THE WELL-WOMAN COOKBOOK

The Well-Woman Cookbook

Patricia Panahi

Kroshka Books
Commack, New York

Editorial Production: Susan Boriotti
Office Manager: Annette Hellinger
Graphics: Frank Grucci and John T'Lustachowski
Information Editor: Tatiana Shohov
Book Production: Donna Dennis, Patrick Davin, Christine Mathosian, Tammy Sauter and Diane Sharp
Circulation: Maryanne Schmidt
Marketing/Sales: Cathy DeGregory

Library of Congress Cataloging-in-Publication Data

Panahi, Patricia.
    The Well-Woman Cookbook, by Patricia Panahi.
        p.   cm.
    ISBN 1-56072-343-2
    1.Women--Health and Hygiene. 2. Vegetarian Cookery. I. Title
RA778.P263   1998   98-33851
613.2'62'08—dc21   CIP

Copyright © 1998 by Patricia Panahi
    Kroshka Books, a division of
    Nova Science Publishers, Inc.
    6080 Jericho Turnpike, Suite 207
    Commack, New York 11725
    Tele. 516-499-3103 Fax 516-499-3146
    e-mail: Novascience@earthlink.net
    e-mail: Novascil@aol.com
    Web Site: http://www.nexusworld.com/nova

All rights reserved. No part of this book may be reproduced, stored in a retrieval system or transmitted in any form or by any means: electronic, electrostatic, magnetic, tape, mechanical photocopying, recording or otherwise without permission from the publishers.

The authors and publisher haven taken care in preparation of this book, but make no expressed or implied warranty of any kind and assume no responsibility for any errors or omissions. No liability is assumed for incidental or consequential damages in connection with or arising out of information contained in this book.

This publication is designed to provide accurate and authoritative information with regard to the subject matter covered herein. It is sold with the clear understanding that the publisher is not engaged in rendering legal or any other professional services. If legal or any other expert assistance is required, the services of a competent person should be sought. FROM A DECLARATION OF PARTICIPANTS JOINTLY ADOPTED BY A COMMITTEE OF THE AMERICAN BAR ASSOCIATION AND A COMMITTEE OF PUBLISHERS.

Printed in the United States of America

To my loving husband, Mark, for his patience and support, his beautiful artwork, and his willingness to sample every recipe in this book.

CONTENTS

Preface .... *xiii*

Introduction *3*

Food For The Body *5*

   1. The Necessary Nutrients 5

   2. Food Review 10

   3. Calcium Robbers 12

Soups & Salads *13*

   Buckwheat Noodle Salad 15

   Steamed Green Salad With Dijon Mustard Sauce 16

   Light Fruit Salad 17

   Green Papaya Salad 18

   Cucumber Tomato Salad 19

   Tofu Salad 20

   Seaweed Salad 21

   Light Pasta Salad 22

   Garden Green Salad 23

   Couscous Salad 25

Sesame-Miso Bean Soup	26
Spinach Potato Soup	27
Cool Yogurt Soup	28
Whole Grain Soup	29
Root Soup	30
Persian Noodle Soup	31
Fresh Garden Soup	33
Middle Eastern Bean Soup	35
Barley Miso Soup	36
Yogurt Vegetable Soup	37

Main Entrees *39*

Cou Cou	41
Lima-Dill Pilaf	43
Whole Grain Stew	44
Mushroom Kale Quiche	46
Cranberry Walnut Sauce	47
Tostada Towers	48
Seitan Stroganoff	50
Zucchini Bake	51
Japanese Vegetable Pancakes	53
New England Potato Pie	55
Stuffed Acorn Squash	57
Lentil Raisin Pilaf	59
Seaweed Sauté	60
Persian Dolmas	61

Black Bean Tamale Pie	63
Celery Sauté	64
Marinated Meatless Steak	65
Jeweled Rice	66
Giant Meatballs	67
Herb Pasta With Tofu Cream Sauce	69
Spiced Millet	70
Macaroni & Beans	71
Herbed Rice With Lemon Broiled Tempeh	72
Seitan Garden Stew	74
Cabbage Pilaf	75
Fresh Herb Sauté	76
Stuffed Eggplant, Green Pepper, And Tomato	77
Spinach Prune Stew	79
Carrot Pilaf	80
Korean Mung Bean Pancakes	81
Chinese Stir Fry	82
Spinach & Eggs	83
Swedish Wheatballs	84
Tofu Tacos	86
Fettuccini Light	87
Burdock Burgers	88
Egyptian Bean Medley	90
Green Bean Pilaf	92
Sausage & Sauerkraut	93

Nutloaf With Mushroom Gravy 94

Green Beans & Eggs 96

Broccoli Cauliflower Casserole 97

Rice & Black-Eyed Peas 98

Stuffed Spinach Mushroom Loaf..99

Potato Tomato Rice 100

Steamed Veggie Basket..101

Pizza Verde..103

Sauces, Snacks, And Side Dishes *105*

Sweet Potato Bake...107

Root Roast...108

Nishimi Vegetables 109

Stuffed Potatoes...110

Rice Balls..111

Tofu Sushi...113

Sautéed Greens..115

Fresh Herb Roll-Up...116

Yogurt-Cucumber Sauce..117

Spinach & Yogurt..118

Beets & Yogurt..119

Yogurt Cheese With Shallots 120

Tahina..121

Lentil Pate' 122

Garbanzo Spread...123

Fava Bean Dip 124

Tofu Almond Spread 125
Homemade Seitan (Wheat Gluten) 126
Tofu Garlic Herb Dip 127
Oriental Dressing 128
Miso Dressing 129
Yogurt Herb Dressing 130
Lemon Dressing 131
Herb Vinegar Dressing 132
Avocado Dressing 133
Avocado Spread 134
Tofu Vanilla Sauce 135
On The Side 136

Drinks and Desserts *137*
Cranberry Spritzer 139
Cranberry Punch 140
Pineapple Spritzer 141
Lime Cooler 142
Yogurt Cooler 143
Watermelon Juice 144
Evening Tea 145
Indian Ginger Tea (Chai) 146
Hibiscus Ginger Ice Tea 147
Cantaloupe Smoothie 148
Banana Yogurt Smoothie 149
Hawaiian Sorbet 150

Pumpkin Pudding	151
Quinoa Pudding	152
Figgy Pudding	153
Tropical Rice Pudding	154
Apricot Couscous Pie	155
Fresh Strawberry Delight	156
Carob Cream Pie	157
Munchies	158
A Final Note	*159*
Tips	160
Glossary	*161*
Bibliography	*165*

Preface

Menopause is upon us. We, the baby boom generation, now have available opportunities that were literally unheard of by previous generations. With a wealth of information at our fingertips, we can approach The Change of Life with knowledge, understanding, and care. As we learn and grow together, and share of our experiences, we can both support each other, and nurture ourselves through this major life transition. This opens up new doors and possibilities that can help us make clear, informative decisions about our bodies, our mental and emotional well-being, and our lives.

With information and understanding, we will be able to make our relationship with our health practitioners a cooperative venture rather than one of dependency. As we become more aware of the choices available to us, we can make wise decisions that will best suit our individual needs.

Nurturing our bodies with healthy, healing foods is a simple, yet very effective step we can take towards easing our transition through menopause. In the pages of this book, I will share with you what I have learned on my journey, along with a delicious, wholesome array of recipes I have either adapted or created to nurture myself through this major life change.

We now have the opportunity and the resources to take control of our lives, understand our bodies, share our wisdom, and view this new phase of life as an opportunity for explorations and creativity, in opening into a land of unexplored possibilities. Let us, as a generation of women, go hand in hand to redefine this stage of life to one of wholeness, flourishing creativity, wisdom, and dignity.

May your PASSAGE be an awakening of your soul.

Patricia Panahi

INTRODUCTION

A major key to obtaining and sustaining optimum health is the food we eat. As we provide our bodies with natural, low fat, high nutrient foods free of refined flour and sugar, hormones, antibiotics, additives, pesticides, and chemical fertilizers, the body responds with health and vitality. Energy is restored. The immune system is enhanced. Balance and harmony returns.

Although there are various other factors involved , such as stress levels, environmental pollution, levels of physical activity, and the degree of previous abuse that will obviously affect our well being, I have found that modifying our diets can be a major step towards revitalizing our bodies and achieving optimum health. It is also a step that just about anyone is capable of taking.

Within the pages of this book I will share with you over 100 wholesome, delicious vegetarian recipes with an array of tastes and textures that are both pleasing to the palate and nurturing to the soul. Although these recipes are suitable for anyone, I have created or adapted them to specifically meet the nutritional needs of a woman.

Nurture yourself with the creamy texture of Miso Tahini Bean Soup. Quench your thirst with the light taste of Pineapple Spritzer. Tantalize your taste buds with exotic Cranberry Walnut Sauce over basmati rice. Entertain family and friends with the new taste sensations of Persian Dolmas, Mushroom Kale Quiche, and Jeweled Rice. These are but a few of the wide variety of healthy, scrumptious dishes you will find.

As women, we now have both the opportunity and the know how to take control of our lives, nurture ourselves, and ignite the spark of vitality and creativity.

Changing our diets is but a step in this journey of self-discovery.

May your journey be an awakening of your soul.

With Love,

Patricia Panahi

Food for the Body

1. The Necessary Nutrients

Most physicians and nutritionists agree that the best way to get the necessary nutrients into the body is through natural, wholesome food. On the other hand, some health practitioners feel that a healthy diet should also be supplemented due to our depleted and overused soil. As individual needs may vary, consult your health practitioner before using supplements. Remember that vitamins and minerals work synergistically, not in isolation.

The following nutrients, listed with some of their sources, are reported to be necessary for a healthy body.

Vitamin A (Beta Carotene)

Helps heart, vision, skin, and bones. Protects against pollution, prevents vaginal dryness, and slows the aging process. Beta carotene, a vitamin A precursor, is an anti-oxidant with cancer fighting properties.

Sources: Green leafy vegetables such as Swiss chard, beet greens, spinach, kale, parsley, watercress, and broccoli. Yellow and orange vegetables and fruit, such as squash, sweet potatoes, carrots, cantaloupe, and apricots. Seaweeds, eggs, and garlic.

Vitamin B Complex

Helps nerves, liver, skin, eyes, and digestion. Produces energy, keeps body resistant to disease, and assists the formation of red blood cells.

Sources: *B_1 (Thiamin):* Brown rice, dried beans, prunes, raisins, nuts, soybeans, wheat germ, lima beans, peas, broccoli, whole grains, seaweed, and eggs.

B_2 (Riboflavin): Beans, spinach, yogurt, whole grains, mushrooms, peas, and eggs.

B_3 (Niacin): Corn flour, carrots, broccoli, whole wheat, tomatoes, cabbage, eggs, and bee pollen.

B_5 (Pantothenic Acid): Whole grains, dark leafy green vegetables, beans, and eggs.

B_6 (Pyridoxine): Brewer's yeast, carrots, peas, spinach, walnuts, wheat germ, sunflower seeds, eggs, avocados, bananas, prunes, and lentils.

B_{12} (Cyanocobalamin): Eggs, nutritional yeast, spirulina.

Biotin: Whole grains, soy beans, green leafy vegetables, and eggs.

Folic Acid: Brown rice, barley, lentils, split peas, dark green leafy vegetables, root vegetables, and brewer's yeast.

Vitamin C

Helps bones, immune system, heart, adrenal and thyroid glands, gums, and rapid healing.

Reduces stress, protects against pollution and infection, wards off cancer, reduces headaches, night sweats, and hot flashes. This vitamin cannot be produced by the body.

Sources: Fresh fruits such, as citrus, strawberries, pineapples, papayas, cantaloupe, and tomatoes. Fresh vegetables, such as broccoli, cauliflower, sweet peppers, green peas, potatoes, cabbage, and onions. Leafy greens, such as parsley, watercress, turnip greens, Swiss chard, and kale.

Vitamin D

Helps calcium and phosphorus absorption, bones, heart, muscles, and immune system. Prevents osteoporosis and cancer, regulates glucose metabolism, reduces risk of adult onset diabetes, and helps prevent tooth decay.
Sources: Sunlight, egg yolks

Vitamin E

Helps heart, circulation, athletic performance, and healing. Prevents cancer, repairs tissue, retards the aging process, reduces hot flashes, prevents vaginal dryness, lessens wrinkles, and treats premenstrual syndrome and lumpy breasts.
Sources: Cold pressed vegetable oils, wheat germ, whole grains, dark leafy greens, nuts, seeds, legumes, and eggs.

Vitamin K

Helps liver, nerves, and normal blood clotting. Reduces menstrual flooding, and may help prevent osteoporosis.
Sources: Green leafy vegetables, yogurt, egg yolk, blackstrap molasses, kelp, alfalfa, green tea.

Bioflavanoids

Helps circulation, heart, blood vessels, and nerves. Lowers cholesterol, fights bacteria, prevents cataracts, reduces hot flashes and water retention, and relieves anxiety.
Sources: Citrus fruit (pulp and rind), dark-red berries, buckwheat, green pepper, and prunes.

Calcium

Helps bones, heart, muscles, nerves, and brain function. Reduces mood swings and bloating, lowers blood pressure, regulates normal blood clotting, and speeds all healing processes. The body cannot produce calcium.

Sources: Seaweeds, yogurt, carob, sesame tahini, leafy green vegetables, blackstrap molasses, tofu precipitated with calcium chloride, figs, nuts & seeds, whole grains, beans.

Magnesium

Helps heart, bones, calcium metabolism, and cell building. Relieves anxiety and fatigue, prevents muscle cramps and depression, assists in the synthesis of proteins, and regulates the acid-alkaline balance of the body.

Sources: Seaweeds, green leafy vegetables, alfalfa, almonds, sunflower seeds, whole grains, potatoes, corn, squash, celery, figs, soy beans, and blackstrap molasses.

Phosphorus

Helps bones, teeth, cell growth, heart, and kidneys. Increases energy, and assists in metabolizing fats and carbohydrates. Phosphorus must be in balance with calcium.

Sources: Eggs, dried beans and peas, whole grains, seeds, nuts, brewer's yeast, dried fruit, and green leafy vegetables.

Essential Fatty Acids

Helps heart, nerves, bones, and endocrine glands. Regulates hormones, maintains immune system, and helps prevent heart disease.

Sources: Flax seeds, pumpkin seeds, sesame seeds, flax seed oil, wheat germ oil, canola oil, sesame oil.

Iron

Helps nerves, energy, immune system, and blood. Produces hemoglobin in the blood which carries oxygen to other parts of the body. Assists in reducing menstrual flooding, headaches, hot flashes, and night sweats.

Sources: Eggs, beets, kelp, blackstrap molasses, sesame seeds, dried beans, leafy green vegetables, pumpkin, dried fruits, and whole grains.

Selenium

Helps heart, pancreas, vision, hair, nails, teeth, immune system, vaginal tissue lubrication, and liver. A potent antioxidant, selenium inhibits the formation of free radicals and may help in decreasing the risk of breast cancer.
Sources: Yogurt, seaweed, garlic, wheat germ, brewer's yeast, eggs.

Boron

Helps bones and calcium metabolism.
Sources: Organic fruits, vegetables, nuts, whole grains, and honey.

Iodine

Helps thyroid gland and liver. Reduces breast lumps, metabolizes fat, and reduces fatigue.
Sources: Seaweed, especially kelp, sea salt, celery, and parsley.

Manganese

Helps bones, nerves, immune system, mammary glands, blood sugar regulation, and fat and protein metabolism.
Sources: Seaweeds, avocados, whole grains, nuts and seeds.

Zinc

Helps digestion, bones, nerves, skin, sex drive, healing of wounds and burns, and energy.
Sources: Eggs, seaweed, pumpkin seeds, blackstrap molasses, wheat germ.

Copper

Helps bones, red blood cells, hemoglobin, fertility, nerves, and skin color. It also assists the body in fighting infection and retaining calcium in the bones.

Sources: Soybeans, seaweeds, almonds, leafy green vegetables, and blackstrap molasses.

2. Food Review

Plant Foods: Most health practitioners agree that a health-supporting diet should be primarily based on whole grains, beans, vegetables, fruits, nuts, and seeds. As there is currently some concern over the use of pesticides and chemical fertilizers in commercial farming, organic produce and grains are advised.

Dairy: While the traditional view is to recommend regular use of dairy products, especially milk, to women, others, such as Susan M. Lark, M.D., suggest avoiding all dairy products due to "...the many negative health aspects"(46) of using them. Dr. Lark recommends alternative sources of calcium such as green leafy vegetables, sesame seeds, and soy beans.

Nutritionist Ann Louise Gittleman suggests the use of nonfat yogurt in her Prime-time diet (167). Yogurt with live cultures helps replace beneficial bacteria in the colon that have been depleted by the use of antibiotics. Note that not all yogurt contains live cultures. Read labels. I prefer to use yogurt from dairy farms that do not use antibiotics or hormones.

Eggs: Eggs are a good source of protein, vitamins B, D, K and zinc. On the other hand, egg yolks are high in fat and cholesterol. With a primarily plant-based diet, I use fertile free-range eggs in moderation. Egg whites may also be used.

Fish, Poultry, and Meat: "Fish and poultry should be eaten more frequently," claims Dr. Lark (60). She recommends reducing meat consumption and increasing grains and vegetables for optimal health.

In her Prime Time Diet, Nutritionist Anne Louise Gittleman advises women to increase their consumption of poultry, fish, beans, legumes, and soy protein (143).

Being a vegetarian, I do not include any meat dishes in my recipes, yet they can be easily modified to accommodate women who prefer to include poultry and fish in their diet. Chicken stock can replace vegetable broth; boneless chicken can be used instead of tofu, tempeh, or Seitan (wheat gluten). Many of the rice recipes and side dishes also go well with broiled fish or chicken. TVP (texturized vegetable protein) can be substituted by ground turkey.

Oils & Fats: While there is no question that a low-fat diet is health supporting for any age group, a NON-FAT diet is not recommended for women. Margarine, although made from plant sources, is not considered a healthy fat as its molecular structure changes during the hydrogenation process. Use healthy fats such as extra virgin olive oil, canola oil, sesame oil, and flaxseed oil. (Flaxseed oil should not be cooked or heated. Use unrefined expeller pressed oils only).

Salt: According to Susan Lark, M.D., "...salt can worsen high blood pressure, bloating and fluid retention, and can contribute to osteoporosis" (43). Lark suggests seasoning food with herbs, spices, garlic, and lemon juice. In addition to these, I tend to use low sodium soy sauce and Bragg liquid aminos for flavoring. These condiments provide flavoring with much less sodium chloride than regular table salt.

Source	Amount	Approx. Sodium Content
Table Salt	1 tsp	2000 mg
Tamari	1 tsp	320 mg
Low sodium Tamari	1 tsp	234 mg
Bragg Liquid Aminos	1 tsp	220 mg

Sugar: Simple sugars are quickly absorbed into the bloodstream and tend to upset the body chemistry. Studies have shown that the consumption of sugar "reduced the level of phosphorous" and caused an increase in the urinary excretion of zinc. It also inhibits the absorption of calcium. (Appleton-37) Even natural sugars such as maple syrup and honey are still sugars, and act similarly. Nevertheless, I have created some nutritious desserts using natural sugars to appease the OCCASIONAL sweet tooth.

3. Calcium Robbers

The following items tend to either inhibit the absorption of calcium, or cause the depletion of this mineral from the body.

Too much protein

Too much phosphorous (sodas)

Refined flour

Processed foods

Refined sugar

Alcohol

Caffeine

Cigarettes

Salt

Aluminum (cookware, baking powder, pickles and relish, toothpaste, and deodorant)

Too much oxalic acid (spinach, rhubarb, chocolate, beet, chard, asparagus)

SOUPS & SALADS

Buckwheat Noodle Salad

WITH IT'S MILD FLAVOR ARAME IS A GREAT INTRODUCTION TO MINERAL RICH SEAWEEDS.

Ingredients

1 cup Arame or Hijiki seaweed, dried (looks like tangled black strings)
1 package buckwheat soba (Japanese noodles)
2 cups lettuce, shredded
2 cup dandelion greens, or other greens of your choice, chopped
1 cup cabbage, shredded
1 cup mung bean sprouts
2 green onions, chopped

Dressing

2 tbsp rice vinegar
1 1/2 tbsp low sodium tamari soy sauce
2 tbsp honey or maple syrup
2 tbsp sesame tahini
1/3 cup water

Directions

1. Soak Arame seaweed in cold water for 30 minutes. Strain and rinse.
2. Cook noodles according to package directions. Strain and rinse.
3. Blend rice vinegar, soy sauce, honey, sesame tahini, and water.
4. On a platter, make a bed of lettuce, dandelion greens, and cabbage.
5. Top with noodles, drained seaweed, mung bean sprouts, and green onions.
6. Add dressing and enjoy for a light lunch or dinner.

Seaweeds are a valuable source of trace minerals

Steamed Green Salad With Dijon Mustard Sauce

TRY GETTING YOUR CALCIUM NATURALLY WITH THIS TANGY LIGHT SALAD.

Ingredients

6 cups greens, chopped (kale, collard, chard, amaranth, or lambs quarter)
1 tbsp sesame seeds

Dressing

1/4 cup lemon juice
1/4 cup water
1 tbsp Dijon mustard
1 clove garlic, minced
2 tbsp Bragg liquid aminos or low sodium tamari soy sauce
1 tbsp sesame tahini

Directions

1. Steam greens for 10-15 minutes or until tender. Let slightly cool.
2. Blend dressing ingredients till smooth. Serve over greens.
3. Garnish with sesame seeds.
4. Serves four.

Greens are a wonderful source of vitamins, minerals, and chlorophyll.

Light Fruit Salad

GREAT FOR HOT WEATHER LIGHT LUNCH

Ingredients

1 cup grapes, seedless
2 apples, sliced
2 pears, sliced
2 bananas, sliced
chopped nuts (optional)
nutmeg (optional)

Dressing

1 cup plain nonfat yogurt
1 cup applesauce
2 ripe bananas

Directions

1. Place fruit in individual serving dishes.
2. Blend dressing ingredients and spoon onto fruit. Garnish with nuts and a sprinkle of nutmeg.

Suggestions

If you prefer a sweeter dressing, add maple syrup, rice syrup, or another sweetener of your choice.
This dish is also good as a dessert.
Use other fruit combinations of your choice.

Fresh organic fruit is packed with essential vitamins and free of fat.

Green Papaya Salad

THIS IS A POPULAR SALAD FROM THAILAND

Ingredients

1 green papaya, coarsely grated or cut in peelings
1 lg tomato, chopped
1 cucumber, chopped
1/2 cup cilantro, coarsely chopped
2 green onions, chopped
1/3 cup roasted almonds or peanuts, chopped

Dressing

2 tbsp sesame oil, roasted
1 tbsp low sodium tamari soy sauce
1 clove garlic, crushed
2 limes, juiced

Directions

1. Mix all ingredients and toss with dressing.
2. Serves four.

Papaya contains enzymes that help digestion.

Cucumber Tomato Salad

A GREAT SIDE DISH FOR RICE

Ingredients

2 cucumbers, chopped
1 lg tomato, chopped
1/2 sm red onion, chopped
1 tbsp parsley, chopped (optional)

Dressing

1 tbsp extra virgin olive oil
2 tbsp lime juice
1/2 tsp sea salt (optional)

Directions

1. Toss all ingredients and serve with a rice or other grain dish.
2. Serves four.

Cucumbers help balance hormones.

Tofu Salad

GREAT AS A DIP, SPREAD, STUFFED IN A TOMATO, OR SERVED ON A BED OF LETTUCE.

Ingredients

1 lb tofu, drained
2 pickles, chopped
20 green olives, chopped
2 tbsp parsley, chopped
1 sm carrot, grated
2 tbsp lemon juice
1 tbsp extra virgin olive oil
3 tbsp soy mayonnaise
1/2 tsp kelp powder
1 tsp mustard
Bragg liquid aminos to taste (optional)

Directions

1. Press tofu to remove excess moisture and pat dry. Crumble into a bowl and mix in remaining ingredients. Chill and serve on a bed of lettuce.
2. Serves six.

Suggestions

May also be served with whole grain crackers, pita bread, raw cut vegetables, or as a sandwich spread. Blend until smooth if using as a dip.

Soy is the most complete plant protein.

Seaweed Salad

SAVOR THE FLAVOR OF THE SEA WITH THE MILD TASTE OF ARAME.

Ingredients

1 cup arame seaweed
1/4 lb green beans, French cut (lengthwise)
2 carrots, julienned
1 tbsp sesame seeds, roasted
2 green onions, chopped

Dressing

1 tbsp rice vinegar
1 tbsp low sodium tamari soy sauce
1 tbsp maple syrup
1 tbsp sesame oil
1 tbsp water

Directions

1. Soak seaweed in cold water for 15-20 minutes. Drain.
2. Steam green beans and carrots for 10 minutes. Let cool.
3. Mix seaweed, green beans, carrots, green onions, and sesame seeds in a bowl.
4. Add dressing and toss. Chill until ready to serve.
5. Serves four.

Arame seaweed is rich in iron and calcium.

Light Pasta Salad

GREAT FOR PICNICS, SNACKS, AND LIGHT LUNCHES

Ingredients

2 cups whole grain pasta spirals, shells, or elbows (tri-color)
1 cup green peas, cooked al dente
10 black olives, sliced
1/2 cup cilantro, coarsely chopped
1/2 sm red onion, chopped (optional)

Dressing

1/2 cup plain nonfat yogurt
2-3 tbsp soy mayonnaise
1 tbsp lime juice
1 tbsp low sodium tamari soy sauce
1 tsp mustard

Directions

1. Cook pasta until al dente (cooked, but firm). Drain and rinse well.
2. Set aside to cool.
3. In large bowl, mix all ingredients well. Chill and serve.
4. Serves six.

Suggestions

If serving as a light lunch, try adding chopped carrots and green pepper for extra vitamins.

Yogurt is a rich source of calcium without the fat.

Garden Green Salad

SERVE THIS SALAD ON A REGULAR BASIS TO PROVIDE
THE BODY WITH "LIVE" FOOD.

Ingredients

Choose one or more from each category:

Greens:
- Lettuce (any kind)
- Green chard (hard stems removed)
- Collards
- Beet Tops
- Turnip Greens
- Mustard greens
- Dandelion greens
- Escarole
- Mixed Salad Greens (packaged)
- Other greens of your choice.

Sprouts:
- Alfalfa
- Radish
- Sunflower
- Buckwheat
- Mung bean

Vegetables:
- Green pepper, chopped or sliced thinly
- Carrots, chopped or in peelings
- Cabbage, shredded (red or green)
- Cucumber, thinly sliced
- Tomato, thinly sliced

Zucchini, thinly sliced or shredded
Yellow summer squash, thinly sliced or shredded
Daikon, thinly sliced or shredded
Beet, shredded
Chinese pea pods
Red or Maui onions, chopped or thinly sliced

Seeds:
Sunflower
Pumpkin
Sesame, roasted

Herbs:
(leaves only)
Parsley
Cilantro
Basil
Mint

Dressing

Choose any of the dressings from chapter five.

Suggestions

Vary the ingredients and dressing, and have a fresh salad daily.

Enjoy fresh vegetables, greens, and herbs regularly for health and vitality.

Couscous Salad

COUSCOUS IS A SMALL WHEAT PASTA POPULAR IN THE MIDDLE EAST.

Ingredients

1 cup whole wheat couscous
1 1/4 cup hot water
1 cup green peas, cooked al dente
1/2 sweet red pepper, chopped
1/2 red onion, chopped
1/3 cup parsley, chopped
2 tbsp extra virgin olive oil
3 tbsp fresh lime juice
1 tbsp Bragg liquid aminos (optional)

Directions

1. In small pot, add couscous to hot water. Bring to a boil. Lower heat and simmer, covered, for about 3 minutes. Remove from heat and let sit for ten minutes or until all moisture is absorbed. Set aside to cool.
2. Add remaining ingredients and mix well. Chill and serve.
3. Serves four.

Suggestions

Try adding chopped green pepper or celery for an extra crunch.

Pasta supplies the body with complex carbohydrates which provide energy.

Sesame-Miso Bean Soup

A CALCIUM-RICH CREAMY SOUP; A MEAL IN ITSELF.

Ingredients

3 shiitake mushrooms, dried
1 cup mixed beans, soaked overnight
1 piece kombu seaweed
1 small onion, shopped
2 cloves garlic, minced
1 bay leaf
1 tsp sage
8 cups water
3-4 tbsp light miso paste
3-4 tbsp sesame tahini

Directions

1. Soak shiitake mushrooms in hot water for 10 minutes
2. Remove hard stems and chop
3. In large pot, cook all ingredients except miso and tahini over low flame until beans are tender, about 1 hour.
4. In blender, mix miso and tahini with some of the bean broth.
5. Stir into bean soup and serve with whole grain bread and a fresh green salad.
6. Serves six.

Suggestions

Add 2 tbsp wakame seaweed, soaked for 10 minutes in hot water, for additional minerals.

Kombu seaweed makes beans more digestible

Spinach Potato Soup

SIMPLE TO MAKE; PACKED WITH NUTRITION

Ingredients

4 potatoes, peeled and quartered
1 onion, chopped
2 cloves garlic, minced
1 bay leaf
1 tbsp rosemary, dried (or 1/3 cup fresh, finely chopped)
1 tsp garden sage
Dash of cayenne (optional)
5 cups vegetable broth
2 cups rice or soy milk
1 lb spinach, finely chopped
2-3 limes
Bragg liquid aminos to taste (optional)

Directions

1. Simmer potatoes, onion, garlic, bay leaf and herbs in broth until potatoes are tender, 15-20 minutes.
2. Remove bay leaf and blend soup until smooth.
3. Add rice milk and bring to a boil.
4. Lower heat and add spinach. Simmer for a few minutes until spinach wilts.
5. Season with lime and serve with warm whole grain bread.
6. Serves six - eight.

Suggestion

Green chard also works well with this recipe.

Spinach is a good source of iron in addition to other minerals.

Cool Yogurt Soup

REFRESHING AND LIGHT FOR A HOT SUMMER DAY

Ingredients

2 cups plain nonfat yogurt
1 lg cucumber, finely chopped
2 green onions, chopped
1 tbsp fresh dill weed, finely chopped
1 tsp dried mint
1/4 cup raisins
1/4 cup walnuts (optional)
1 tsp sea salt (optional)
1 cup cold water
Ice as needed
Flat bread such as Lavosh or tortilla (optional)

Directions

1. In medium bowl, stir yogurt until creamy.
2. Mix in cucumber, green onions, dill weed, mint, raisins, walnuts, and salt.
3. Add cold water and stir. Pour into individual serving dishes with one or more ice cubes in each bowl.
4. Toast bread till crispy. Crumble into soup.

Suggestions

This cooling soup is best served VERY cold. Add the flat bread to make it a light meal.

Yogurt is cooling to an overheated body

Whole Grain Soup

A HEARTY SOUP THAT'S A MEAL IN ITSELF.

Ingredients

1 pkg *Kashi (whole grain cereal)
1 onion, chopped
1 burdock root, thinly sliced
8 cups vegetable broth
4 shiitake mushrooms, dried, soaked in hot water
1 cup parsley, chopped
Bragg liquid aminos to taste (optional)
3-4 limes

Directions

1. In large pot, combine Kashi, onion, burdock root, and broth.
2. Bring to a boil. Lower flame and simmer.
3. Remove hard stems from mushrooms and chop.
4. Add to soup and cook over low flame for 30-45 minutes or until grains are well cooked. Add extra water if soup becomes too thick.
5. Mix in parsley and season with Bragg and lime.
6. Serves six - eight.

Suggestions

This soup works well in a crock pot. Let simmer all day and add parsley just before serving.

Whole grains are high in fiber which may help prevent colon cancer.

Root Soup

A SIMPLE CONCOCTION OF MINERAL RICH ROOTS.

Ingredients

1 rutabaga, cubed
1 onion, chopped
2 cloves garlic, minced
1/2 tsp sage, dried
1/4 tsp savory, dried
1/4 tsp thyme, dried
6 cups vegetable stock
2 potatoes, cubed
3 carrots, chopped
1 turnip, cubed
1/2 cup parsley, chopped
Bragg liquid aminos to taste (optional)
3-4 limes

Directions

1. In large pot, combine rutabaga, onion, garlic, herbs and vegetable stock.
2. Bring to a boil. Lower flame and cook for 15-20 minutes.
3. Add potatoes, carrots, and turnip.
4. Simmer for another 15-20 minutes or until vegetables are tender.
5. Add parsley and season with Bragg and lime.
6. Serve with whole grain bread and fresh green salad.
7. Serves six.

Rutabagas and turnips are sources of calcium.

Persian Noodle Soup

THIS IS A TRADITIONAL ALL-TIME FAVORITE.

Ingredients

1 cup garbanzo beans, cooked
1 cup red kidney beans, cooked
1/2 cup lentils
1 tsp tumeric
8 cups vegetable broth
1 bunch spinach, chopped
2 bunches parsley, chopped
2 bunches cilantro, chopped
1 bunch green onions, green part only, chopped
1/3 pkg soba (Japanese noodles), broken in half
2 tbsp whole wheat flour
1/2 cup whey or 1-2 cups yogurt
1 cup water
2 onions, chopped
2 tbsp sesame or canola oil
1 tbsp mint, dried

Directions

1. In large pot, bring garbanzo beans, kidney beans, lentils, turmeric, and vegetable broth to a boil. Lower flame and simmer for 20 minutes or until lentils are cooked.
2. Add spinach, parsley, cilantro, green onions and noodles. Simmer for 5-10 minutes.
3. Mix flour with water and whey. (If using yogurt, add after serving and reduce water to 1/2 cup). Stir into soup and simmer, stirring occasionally until soup has thickened.

4. Sauté onion in sesame oil until brown and translucent. Mix in dried mint.
5. Serve soup in large bowl topped with onion/mint mixture.
6. Serves eight.

Kidney beans lend support to the kidneys.

Fresh Garden Soup

SAVOR THE BOUNTY OF SUMMER VEGETABLES WITH THIS DELICIOUS SOUP SIMMERED IN A LIGHT BROTH WITH FRESH HERBS.

Ingredients

3 shiitake mushrooms, dried
3 potatoes, cubed
3 carrots, sliced
1/4 lb green beans, chopped
1 sm onion, chopped
2 cloves garlic, minced
1 bay leaf
1 tbs fresh sage, chopped (or 1 tsp dried)
1 tbsp fresh thyme, chopped (or tsp dried)
8 cups vegetable broth
1 zucchini, chopped
1 yellow summer squash, chopped
1 cup whole grain pasta, spirals or shells
1/2 cup tomato sauce
1/3 cup parsley, chopped
2 tbsp kuzu or arrowroot powder
2 lemons, sliced

Directions

1. Soak shiitake mushrooms in hot water for 15 minutes. Drain. Remove hard stem and chop.
2. In large pot, combine mushrooms, potatoes, carrots, green beans, seasonings and broth. Bring to a boil. Reduce heat and simmer for 10 minutes.
3. Add pasta and cook until al dente, 5-8 minutes.

4. Add zucchini and yellow squash to soup. Blend tomato sauce, parsley and kuzu. Mix into soup and simmer, stirring regularly, until slightly thickened.
5. Season individual dishes with a twist of lemon. Serve with whole grain bread. Serves six.

Summer squash is light and easy to digest.

Middle Eastern Bean Soup

WARMING AND NURTURING IN ITS SIMPLICITY.

Ingredients

2 cups pinto beans, soaked overnight
1 piece kombu
1 onion, chopped
2 cloves garlic, minced
6 cups water
3-4 limes
1 tbs extra virgin olive oil
Bragg liquid aminos or tamari soy sauce to taste

Directions

1. Cook beans, kombu, onion, and garlic in water until beans are tender. (1-1 1/2 hrs conventional, 1/2 hr pressure cooker)
2. Remove kombu and discard.
3. Serve soup in individual bowls. Season with lime juice, olive oil, and Bragg liquid aminos. Serve with warm whole wheat pita bread and green salad.
4. Serves eight.

Olive oil, a monounsaturated fat, is the most commonly used oil in traditional Mediterranean cuisine where heart disease is minimal.

Barley Miso Soup

DELIGHTFULLY EASY TO MAKE, YET VERY SOOTHING TO BODY AND SOUL.

Ingredients

1 cup barley pearls
1 onion, chopped
6 cups water
1 carrot, sliced
2 ribs celery, chopped
2 tbsp parsley, chopped
3-4 tbsp light miso paste
1/2 cup water

Directions

1. In large pot, simmer barley and onion in water until barley is well-cooked, about 35-40 minutes.
2. Add carrots, celery and parsley and simmer for another 10 minutes. Stir occasionally to prevent bottom from sticking.
3. Blend miso paste in water. Stir into soup and serve. Add additional miso if needed. Serve with whole grain bread and green salad. Serves four.

Miso strengthens the blood and lymph system. It is also a good source of enzymes, calcium, and iron.

Yogurt Vegetable Soup

THIS IS SIMPLY THAT KIND OF SOUP THAT HEALS ANYTHING. TRY IT IN PLACE OF CHICKEN SOUP NEXT TIME YOU OR A FAMILY MEMBER FEEL "UNDER THE WEATHER".

Ingredients

1 cup garbanzo beans, cooked
1 cup pinto beans, cooked
1/2 cup bulghar (or whole grains, steel cut)
1 tsp tumeric
8 cups vegetable broth
1 onion, chopped
2 carrots, sliced
1 turnip, cubed
2 bunches spinach, chopped
1 bunch parsley, chopped
1 bunch cilantro, chopped
1 bunch green onions, chopped
Plain nonfat yogurt

Directions

1. In large pot, bring beans, bulghar, and broth to a boil. Lower flame and simmer for 30 minutes, stirring occasionally to prevent sticking.
2. Add carrots, and turnips. Simmer for another 15 minutes or until vegetables are cooked.
3. Add spinach, parsley, cilantro, and green onion.
4. Simmer for 5-8 minutes or until greens are tender.
5. Pour into individual serving bowls and top with a dollop of yogurt.
6. Serves eight.

Main Entrees

Cou Cou

A Delicious New Way To Eat Your Greens!

Ingredients

2 cups collard greens or green chard, chopped
2 cups kale, chopped
2 cups leeks, green part only, chopped
1 cup walnut pieces
3 tbsp whole wheat flour
10 egg whites, or 5 lg eggs
1/3 cup dried cranberries (optional)
1 tsp sea salt (optional)
1 tbsp extra virgin olive oil

Directions

1. Wash greens and remove excess water.
2. Add all remaining ingredients except olive oil and mix well.
3. Heat 1/2 tbsp olive oil in non-stick pan.
4. Add mixture and pat down.
5. Cover and cook over medium heat for 5 minutes.
6. Cut into wedges and loosen sides. Drizzle with remaining oil.
7. Wrap lid in paper towel (to absorb excess moisture) and cook over low flame for another ten minutes.
8. Serve with Yogurt-Cucumber Sauce (p. 115) and warm whole wheat pita or tortilla bread.
9. Serves four.

Suggestions

Replace one or all greens with spinach.
Wrap up leftovers in tortilla bread for delicious sandwiches.

Collards and Kale are rich in Calcium and Vitamin C.

Lima-Dill Pilaf

THIS UNIQUE DISH WILL GIVE YOU A NEW APPRECIATION FOR RICE.

Ingredients

1 1/2 cups brown or basmati rice
3 cups vegetable broth
1 cup lima or fava beans, cooked al dente
2/3 cup fresh dill weed, chopped
pinch of saffron, powdered (optional)

Directions

1. Combine all ingredients and bring to a boil.
2. Cover lid with towel and cook over low flame for 30-45 minutes.
3. Serve with Yogurt-Cucumber (p. 115) sauce or plain yogurt.
4. Serves four.

Suggestions

For added protein, sauté 1/2 lb previously frozen cubed tofu or Seitan (wheat gluten) with onions. Add 1 cup vegetable broth and a pinch of tumeric.
Simmer over low flame for 10-15 minutes. Serve over rice.

Soy beans help balance estrogen levels.

Whole Grain Stew

A HEARTY MEAL FOR A COOL WINTER'S EVE;
A GREAT RECIPE FOR THE CROCKPOT.

Ingredients

1 kohlrabi, rutabaga, or butternut squash, cubed
1 lg onion, chopped
1-2 tbsp sesame oil
1 1/2 cup garbanzo beans, cooked
1/2 cup yellow split peas
1/3 cup barley pearls
1/3 cup rolled oats
1/3 cup bulgar
1 tsp tumeric, powdered
1 tsp cinnamon, powdered
1/2 tsp allspice, powdered
8 cups vegetable broth
1/2 cup parsley, shopped

Directions

1. Sauté kohlrabi and onion in oil.
2. In large pot, bring garbanzo beans, split peas, barley, oats, bulgar, spices, and broth to a boil.
3. Add kohlrabi and onions. Lower flame and simmer, stirring occasionally, for 35-45 minutes or until vegetables and grains are well-cooked. Add parsley and simmer for another minute.
4. Serve with whole grain bread and green salad.
5. Serves eight.

Suggestions

For reduced fat, add raw kohlrabi and onion directly to stew.
For added protein and texture, sauté 1/2 lb seitan
(wheat gluten) with vegetables.
Season with Bragg liquid aminos.

Mushroom Kale Quiche

ENTERTAIN YOUR FRIENDS WITH THIS HEALTHY VERSION OF A BRUNCH FAVORITE.

Ingredients

1 pre-baked pie crust, whole wheat preferred
1 tbsp extra virgin olive oil
1/2 onion, chopped
2 cloves garlic, minced
6 mushrooms, sliced
2 cups kale, finely chopped
1 lb tofu, drained and pat dry
1/2 cup soy milk
1 tsp dried mustard
1 tsp rosemary, dried
1 tsp thyme, dried
2 tbsp low sodium tamari
1/3 cup feta cheese, crumbled (optional)
2 egg whites

Directions

1. Sauté onion, garlic, and mushrooms in olive oil till tender.
2. Add kale and sauté for a few more minutes until it wilts.
3. Blend tofu, soy milk, mustard, herbs, tamari, Feta, and egg whites.
4. Fold in kale mixture and pour into pie shell.
5. Bake at 350 degrees F for 25-35 minutes or until set.
6. Serves four - six.

Rosemary improves memory and freshens the breath.

Cranberry Walnut Sauce

A UNIQUE, EXOTIC FLAVOR THAT WILL DELIGHT YOUR TASTE BUDS

Ingredients

1 lg onion, finely chopped
1 tbsp canola oil
2 cups walnuts, ground
2 cups cranberry sauce, mashed (home made preferred, sweetened)
1 cup water
2 tbsp lemon juice

Directions

1. Sauté onion in oil until brown.
2. Mix in remaining ingredients.
3. Simmer for 15-20 minutes, stirring occasionally.
4. Serve over a bed of rice, couscous, or millet.
5. Serves four - six.

Tostada Towers

FUN TO EAT AND EASY TO MAKE!

Ingredients

1 1/2 cups black beans, cooked and drained
1 tsp cumin powder
1 tsp garlic powder
1 tsp onion powder
1 tsp low sodium tamari soy sauce
4-6 corn tortillas
Mild salsa or taco sauce
1 avocado, mashed (optional)

Toppings

Plain nonfat yogurt, strained through cheese cloth (overnight)
Shredded lettuce
Greens of your choice, shredded
Green onions, chopped
Tomato, chopped
Black olives, sliced
Cilantro, chopped
Alfalfa sprouts

Directions

1. Mash black beans.
2. Season with cumin, onion powder, garlic powder, and soy sauce.
3. Bake tortillas till crispy.

4. Top with layer of beans, salsa, avocado, and yogurt.

5. Layer with vegetables.
6. Serves four - six.

Alfalfa is one of the richest mineral foods. It is also available in convenient tablet form.

Seitan Stroganoff

YOU WON'T EVEN MISS THE MEAT IN THIS DELIGHTFUL DISH.

Ingredients

1 lb prepared seitan, cubed
1 lg onion, finely chopped
1 clove garlic, minced
1/2 lb mushrooms, chopped
1 tbsp canola oil
3 tbsp wheat flour
1 cup water or vegetable broth
1/2 cup plain nonfat yogurt
2-3 tbsp lemon juice
Bragg liquid aminos to taste (optional)

Directions

1. Heat oil in non-stick pan. Sauté onions till translucent.
2. Add seitan and onions and sauté till golden brown.
3. Add flour and make a roux.
4. Slowly add water, stirring constantly to avoid lumping.
5. Simmer for 5-8 minutes, stirring occasionally, until sauce thickens.
6. Stir in yogurt and lemon juice. Do not boil.
7. Season with Bragg liquid aminos.
8. Serve over a bed of whole grain noodles.
9. Serves four - six.

Seitan is a lowfat source of protein.

Zucchini Bake

BOTH LIGHT AND ELEGANT, THIS DISH WILL GIVE YOU A NEW APPRECIATION FOR THIS SUMMER SQUASH.

Ingredients

2 cups zucchini, grated (about 1 lg or 2 sm zucchini)
1/3 cup whole wheat flour
1/2 cup walnut pieces
2 tsp onion powder
1 tsp garlic powder
1/4 cup fresh basil, chopped (or 1 tbsp dried)
1/2 tsp kelp granules or sea salt (optional)
1/3 cup brewers yeast
8 egg whites, or 4 eggs, beaten
2 tsp extra virgin olive oil

Directions

1. Preheat oven to 350 degrees F.
2. Spread grated zucchini on large platter or tray and lightly press with paper towel to remove excess water.
3. In large bowl, mix all ingredients except olive oil.
4. Brush pie pan or glass baking dish with 1 tsp olive oil.
5. Pour in zucchini mixture and spread evenly.
6. Bake at 350 degrees for 15 minutes.
7. Cut in wedges and loosen sides.
8. Drizzle remaining oil in grooves.
9. Bake for another 15 minutes at same temperature.
10. Serve with warm whole grain bread and fresh salad.
11. Serves four.

Suggestions

Bake in pie crust.
Use one cup yellow summer squash in place of one cup zucchini.

Brewers yeast is an excellent source of B vitamins.

Japanese Vegetable Pancakes

"OKONOMI-YAKI" SHOPS ARE FREQUENTED BY YOUNG JAPANESE WHERE THEY CAN FLIP THEIR PANCAKES ON A GRILL RIGHT AT THEIR TABLE.
ADAPTED FROM A RECIPE CONTRIBUTED BY YASUKO OKUBA

Ingredients

1 1/2 cups whole wheat flour
1 cup water
4 egg whites, or 2 eggs, slightly beaten
1/2 tsp kelp granules or sea salt (optional)
1 tbsp tapioca starch (optional)
1 cup cabbage (packed), finely chopped or shredded
1 cup kale, (packed), finely chopped
1 small carrot, grated
Sesame oil
Nori flakes (optional)

Sauce

2 tbsp low sodium tamari
2 tbsp mirin or maple syrup
3 tbsp rice vinegar
3 tbsp tomato sauce
3 tbsp orange juice
1 tbsp kuzu
1 tbsp water
2 tbsp sherry
4 tbsp water

Directions

Sauce:
1. Mix first five ingredients in blender until smooth.
2. Simmer over low flame.
3. Mix kuzu with 1 tbsp water and add to mixture.
4. Simmer for several minutes, stirring constantly, until slightly thickened.
5. Add sherry and water.
6. Cook a few more minutes and set aside to cool.
7. Sauce may be made ahead of time.

Pancakes:
1. In large bowl, mix flour, water, eggs, kelp, and tapioca starch.
2. Fold in vegetables.
3. Brush griddle with small amount of sesame oil and heat.
4. Cook pancakes for about 4-5 minutes on each side, or until brown.
5. Serve topped with sauce and sprinkled with nori flakes.
6. Serves four.

Suggestions

You may also use your favorite barbecue sauce, sweet and sour sauce, or try prepared Tonkatsu sauce, available in some supermarkets.

Try adding or substituting other vegetables such as chopped spinach, sliced mushrooms, corn kernels, green peas, mung bean sprouts, or other vegetables of your choice.

Cabbage, along with other cruciferous vegetables, is considered a cancer inhibiter.

New England Potato Pie

A HEALTHY VARIATION OF AN OLD-TIME NEW ENGLAND FAVORITE.

Ingredients

1 onion, chopped
1 tbsp extra virgin olive oil
1/2 lb tofu, previously frozen and defrosted
1 tbsp low sodium tamari soy sauce
6 medium potatoes, cooked and mashed
1/2 cup corn kernels, cooked
1 carrot, grated
1/2 cup green peas, cooked al dente
1 tsp kelp powder or granules
4 egg whites, or 2 eggs, beaten
Extra virgin olive oil or flax seed oil (optional)

Directions

1. Sauté onion in olive oil until translucent.
2. Squeeze out excess water from tofu and pat dry.
3. Shred and add to onion mixture along with soy sauce.
4. Sauté a few minutes until tofu begins to slightly brown.
5. Set aside.
6. In large bowl, mix potatoes, corn, carrot, peas, kelp, and eggs.
7. Oil deep dish pie pan.
8. Spread half of the potato mixture across the bottom.
9. Top with a layer of tofu and onion mixture.
10. Add remaining potato mixture and spread evenly.

11. Bake at 350 degrees F for 40-45 minutes.
12. Drizzle with olive or flaxseed oil and serve with a fresh green salad.
13. Serves four - six.

Suggestions

Use 1/2 cup each chopped green and red bell pepper in place of carrots and peas.

Stuffed Acorn Squash

A TASTY ADDITION TO A HOLIDAY FEAST.

Ingredients

1 cup whole wheat couscous
1 1/4 cups vegetable broth
2 tsp sesame oil
1 onion, finely chopped
8 dried apricots, soaked for 1 hour
1 cup walnuts, chopped
1 tsp sage
1 tsp thyme
1 tbsp low sodium tamari soy sauce (optional)
2 large acorn squash
1/2 cup water

Directions

1. Bring vegetable broth to a boil.
2. Mix in couscous.
3. Cover and simmer over very low flame for 3 minutes.
4. Set aside until all liquid is absorbed.
5. Heat sesame oil in nonstick pan.
6. Sauté' onions until translucent.
7. Chop apricots and mix in with onions along with walnuts.
8. Add couscous, herbs, and soy sauce to onion mixture; mix well.
9. Cut acorn squash in half and remove seeds and fibers.
10. Cut top and bottom so that the squash doesn't wobble.

11. Stuff with couscous dressing and place cut sides up in baking dish.
12. Add water and bake, covered, at 350 degrees F, or until squash is tender.
13. Serve with Green Papaya Salad or other salad of your choice.
14. Serves four.

Acorn squash is rich in beta carotene.

Lentil Raisin Pilaf

A COMPLETE PROTEIN DISH THAT WILL MAKE YOU FEEL YOU'RE HAVING DESSERT FIRST!

Ingredients

1 cup brown rice
1/2 cup barley pearls
1/2 cup lentils, cooked
1/2 cup raisins
1 tsp cinnamon
3 cups vegetable broth
1/2 cup almonds, slivered
Bragg liquid aminos to taste (optional)

Directions

1. Wash brown rice and barley.
2. Mix all ingredients except almonds and Bragg; bring to a boil.
3. Lower flame and simmer, covered, for 45 minutes.
4. Lightly toast almonds in oven or non-stick skillet.
5. Fluff rice and mix in almonds.
6. Season with Bragg and serve with Green Papaya or Garden Green salad.
7. Serves four.

Almonds help stimulate a sluggish digestive track.

Seaweed Sauté

WITH A MILD FLAVOR, AND MORE CALCIUM THAN MILK, ARAME SEAWEED IS A WINNER!

Ingredients

1/2 cup arame seaweed or sea palm fronds
3 shiitake mushrooms, dried
1/2 onion, chopped
2 cloves garlic, minced
1 tbsp sesame seed oil
1/2 lb tofu, drained and cubed
2 carrots, julienned
1 burdock root, julienned
1/2 tsp fresh ginger, grated
1 tbsp sesame seeds, roasted
1 tbsp low sodium tamari soy sauce

Directions

1. Soak the arame seaweed in cold water for 15 minutes.
2. Soak the shiitake mushrooms in hot water for 10 minutes.
3. Drain mushrooms, remove hard stems, and cut in thin strips.
4. Steam burdock and carrots till cooked al dente.
5. Sauté' onion and garlic in sesame oil till translucent.
6. Add tofu and mushrooms. Sauté' till tofu is golden.
7. Add carrots, burdock, seaweed, tamari and sesame seeds.
8. Mix to blend flavors.
9. Serve with a cooked grain.
10. Serves four.

Shiitake mushrooms help prevent high blood pressure and lower cholesterol.

Persian Dolmas

A GREAT DISH FOR A PARTY, POTLUCK, PICNIC, OR A LIGHT MEAL.

Ingredients

1 1/2 cups rice
1 1/2 cups vegetable broth
1 cup yellow split peas, cooked al dente
8 green onions, finely chopped
2/3 cup fresh dill weed, chopped
1 bunch chives, chopped
2 tsp savory, dried
2 tsp tumeric
1 cup plain, nonfat yogurt
1 lemon, juiced
2 tbsp Bragg liquid aminos
4 tsp olive oil
1 jar or can grape leaves (if fresh leaves are available, pick tender leaves)
1 cup water

Directions

1. Bring vegetable broth to a boil.
2. Add rice and reduce flame.
3. Cover and simmer for 15 minutes or until liquid is absorbed.
4. Mix rice with split peas, herbs, yogurt, lemon juice, tumeric, Bragg liquid aminos and 2 tsp olive oil.
5. Remove stem from grape leaf and lay flat.
6. Stuff each leaf with about one tablespoon of mixture and fold up sides.
7. Place extra leaves on the bottom of a large non-stick pot.

8. Top with layers of stuffed grape leaves.
9. Place a heavy plate on top of the last layer to help keep them in place.
10. Add water, cover, and bring to a boil.
11. Simmer over very low flame for one hour or until leaves are tender and water is absorbed. Add more water if necessary.

Black Bean Tamale Pie

ENJOY A LOWFAT VERSION OF THIS SOUTH-OF-THE-BORDER TREAT.

Ingredients

1 1/2 cups black beans, cooked
1 cup corn kernels
1 sm onion, chopped
1 green pepper, chopped
2 cups tomato juice (organic, bottled)
1 tsp garlic powder
1 1/2 tsp cumin powder
1 cup corn meal
1 tsp baking powder
1/2 cup rice milk
2 egg whites, or 1 egg
1 tbsp canola oil

Directions

1. In large bowl, mix beans, corn, onion, green pepper, tomato juice, garlic powder and cumin.
2. Pour into a 8 1/2 x 8 1/2" baking dish.
3. Mix remaining ingredients and pour on top of bean mixture.
4. Spread evenly. Some of the mixture will disappear into the tomato juice.
5. Bake at 425 degrees F for 20-25 minutes.
6. Serve with some mild salsa, slices of avocado, and a fresh green salad.
7. Serves four - six.

Cumin is antispasmodic and antiviral. It also helps with digestion.

Celery Sauté

THE COOL TASTE OF MINT ADDS A UNIQUE FLAVOR TO THIS LOW-CAL DISH.

Ingredients

1 lg onion, chopped
1 tbsp canola oil
2 cups celery, cut into 1 inch pieces
1 tsp tumeric
1 tbsp low sodium tamari soy sauce
1/2 lb prepared seitan, cubed
1 cup fresh mint, chopped
2 cups fresh parsley, chopped
1/2 cup lime juice (or lemon)
1 cup vegetable broth

Directions

1. Sauté onion in oil till translucent.
2. Add celery along with tumeric and soy sauce; sauté till slightly golden.
3. Stir in seitan, mint, and parsley.
4. Cook for another 3 minutes, stirring constantly.
5. Add lime juice and vegetable broth; bring to a boil.
6. Simmer over low flame for 20-30 minutes or until celery is tender.
7. Serve over a bed of basmati rice.
8. Serves four - six.

Marinated Meatless Steak

A DISH TO APPEASE THE "MEAT AND POTATO" PEOPLE.

Ingredients

1 lb tofu (previously frozen and thawed)

Marinade

1/4 cup low sodium tamari soy sauce
1 tbsp sesame oil
1 tbsp maple syrup
2 cloves garlic, crushed
2 green onions, finely chopped
1 tbsp fresh ginger, grated
1/4 cup sherry (optional)

Directions

1. Use paper towel to press out excess water from tofu.
2. Slice into 1/2 thick "steaks".
3. Mix all marinade ingredients.
4. Marinate tofu for a minimum of one hour (best overnight)
5. Broil or grill until brown on each side.
6. Serve with baked potato and steamed broccoli, or try Root Roast (p. 106).
7. This dish is also good with plain rice.

Ginger stimulates digestion and helps improve circulation.

Jeweled Rice

A Colorful Dish Fit For A Feast

Ingredients

2 cups basmati rice
3 cups vegetable broth
1 cup sugarless orange marmalade
1 cup dried cranberries
1/2 tsp cardamom, freshly ground
1/3 cup almonds, slivered or sliced
1/2 cup pistachios, raw
Flax seed oil (optional)

Directions

1. In medium pot, bring rice and water to a boil.
2. Add marmalade, cranberries, cardamom, and salt.
3. Cover, reduce heat, and simmer for 20-30 minutes.
4. Toast almonds and pistachios in a nonstick skillet or toaster oven.
5. Fluff rice and mix in nuts.
6. Drizzle with flax seed oil.
7. Serve with a side of plain yogurt.
8. Serves four.

Cardamom aids digestion.

Giant Meatballs

SAVOR THIS ADAPTATION OF A TRADITIONAL TURKISH RECIPE FROM THE CAUCASUS MOUNTAINS OF AZARBAYEJAN.

Ingredients

1 1/2 cups TVP
1 cup vegetable broth, hot
1 1/2 cups brown or basmati rice, cooked
1 cup yellow split peas, cooked and mashed
1 cup parsley, chopped
6 green onions, finely chopped
1 tsp savory, dried
1 tbsp Bragg liquid aminos
4 egg whites or 2 eggs
1/2 cup walnut pieces
8 prunes
1 cup vegetable broth

Directions

1. Mix TVP and hot broth. Cover and let stand for ten minutes or until all liquid is absorbed.
2. In large bowl, mix TVP, rice, split peas, parsley, green onions, savory, Bragg liquid aminos, and egg whites.
3. Divide mixture into four sections.
4. Shape each section into a large ball.
5. Push 2 prunes and some walnuts into the middle of each ball and smooth over.
6. Place in large casserole dish with broth.

7. Cover and bake at 350 degrees F for 20-30 minutes or until firm.
8. Serve with green salad.
9. Serves four - six.

Suggestions

This dish may also be made into a Neat Pie by spreading in an oiled pie dish and baking, covered, for 20-25 minutes.

Herb Pasta With Tofu Cream Sauce

A DELICIOUSLY SIMPLE DISH YOU CAN PUT TOGETHER IN NO TIME.

Ingredients

1 onion, chopped
2 cloves garlic, minced
1 tbsp extra virgin olive oil
1/2 lb tofu, drained and pat dry
1/2 cup rice or soy milk
1 tbsp low sodium tamari
3 cups (about 1 lb) whole grain pasta, shells or spirals
1 cup fresh basil, chopped
1/3 cup soy Parmesan or lite Parmesan cheese

Directions

1. Sauté onion and garlic until lightly brown.
2. Blend with tofu, rice milk, and tamari.
3. Cook pasta according to package directions.
4. Toss with basil and mix with tofu sauce.
5. Pour into 8 1/2 x 8 1/2" baking dish and top with Parmesan.
6. Bake at 350 degrees F for 15-20 minutes.
7. Serve with a fresh green salad.
8. Serves four - six.

Garlic helps keep a healthy heart.

Spiced Millet

THIS RECIPE IS COOLING AND HELPS WITH DIGESTION.

Ingredients

1/2 cup millet
1/4 cup mung beans
1 tbsp sesame oil
1 tsp coriander seeds, crushed
1/2 tsp fennel seeds
1 tsp cumin seeds
1 sm butternut squash, peeled and cubed
1/2 tsp tumeric
6 cups water
1/2 tsp sea salt (optional)

Directions

1. Wash millet and mung beans. Set aside.
2. In medium pot, heat oil and add coriander, fennel, and cumin seeds.
3. Sauté for 2 minutes.
4. Add millet, mung beans, vegetables, and tumeric.
5. Sauté for 3-4 minutes.
6. Add water and salt.
7. Bring to a boil; then lower flame.
8. Simmer over low flame, covered, for 1hr.
9. Add extra water if necessary.
10. Serves four - six.

Millet is an alkaline grain. It is helpful when the body has become too acidic.

Macaroni & Beans

TAHINI AND MISO LEND A CREAMY TEXTURE TO THIS NURTURING DISH.

Ingredients

1 onion, chopped
2 cloves garlic, minced
1 tbsp sesame oil
1/2 lb mushrooms, sliced
1 tbs fresh oregano, chopped (or 1 tsp dried)
2 cups whole grain elbow pasta, cooked al dente
2 tbsp light miso
1 1/2 tbsp sesame tahini
1 cup water
1/2 cup aduki beans, cooked
Dash of cayenne (optional)

Directions

1. In large pot, sauté onion and garlic until tender.
2. Add mushrooms and oregano and sauté for a few minutes until tender.
3. Mix in pasta and aduki beans.
4. Blend miso, tahini, and water.
5. Mix with pasta and beans.
6. Season with cayenne.
7. Cook for a few minutes for flavors to blend.
8. Serve with a fresh green salad.
9. Serves four.

Aduki beans are beneficial to the kidneys.

Herbed Rice With Lemon Broiled Tempeh

THE LEMONY TEMPEH WONDERFULLY COMPLEMENTS THE SAVORY HERBS IN THE RICE.

Ingredients

1 1/2 pkg tempeh
3 tbsp extra virgin olive oil
1/3 cup lemon juice
1 tbsp low sodium tamari soy sauce
1 clove garlic, crushed
1/2 small onion, grated
1/2 tsp thyme
1/2 tsp rosemary
1 1/2 cups brown or basmati rice
1 cup parsley, finely chopped
1 cup cilantro, finely chopped
1/2 cup green onions, green part only, finely chopped
1 tsp sea salt (optional)
3 cups water

Directions

1. Steam tempeh for 10 minutes; set aside to cool.
2. Cut into 1 inch cubes.
3. Mix olive oil, lemon juice, soy sauce, garlic, onion, thyme, and rosemary to make marinade.
4. Coat tempeh well and let marinate for at least one hour.
5. Wash rice and add to water along with fresh herbs and sea salt.
6. Bring to a boil.

7. Lower flame and simmer for 35-45 minutes.
8. Bake tempeh for 20 minutes at 325 degrees F.
9. Fluff rice and serve with tempeh.
10. Serves four.

Thyme is antifungal and antibacterial

Seitan Garden Stew

A COMPLETE, WHOLESOME MEAL, ALL IN ONE POT!

Ingredients

1 cup garbanzo beans, cooked
2 onions, chopped
1 lb prepared seitan
3 potatoes, quartered
1/2 lb green beans, French cut (lengthwise)
1 tomato, quartered
1 Japanese eggplant, cut into 1 inch pieces
1 tsp tumeric
1/4 cup lemon juice
4 cups vegetable broth
Bragg liquid aminos to taste (optional)

Directions

1. Mix all ingredients and bring to a boil.
2. Lower flame and simmer until vegetables are well-cooked, about 35-45 minutes.
3. Serve with whole grain flat bread.

Suggestions

Toast flat bread and tear into pieces. Add to stew.

Cabbage Pilaf

THE TASTE OF CABBAGE IS COMPLIMENTED BY MILD SPICES

Ingredients

1 tbsp sesame oil
1 tbsp cumin seeds
1 tsp tumeric
1 onion, chopped
3 cups cabbage, shredded
1 1/2 cups brown or basmati rice
3 cups vegetable broth
1 tsp sea salt (optional)

Directions

1. Heat oil in wok or nonstick pan.
2. Add cumin seeds and tumeric. Stir for one minute.
3. Include onion and sauté till golden.
4. Mix in cabbage and stir fry for another 3-5 minutes.
5. Wash rice and add broth and salt.
6. Bring to a boil; stir in cabbage mixture.
7. Lower heat and cook, covered for 35-45 minutes.
8. Serve with sautéed seitan or tofu and Green Papaya Salad (p.16), or salad of your choice.
9. Serves four.

Fresh Herb Sauté

AROMATIC FRESH HERBS ARE USED AS A MAIN INGREDIENT IN THIS SAVORY ACCOMPANIMENT TO RICE.

Ingredients

1 onion, chopped
1 tbsp canola oil
1/2 lb prepared seitan, cubed
1 tsp tumeric
2 cups parsley, chopped
1 1/2 cups green onion, green part only, finely chopped
1/2 cup fenugreek leaves, chopped (or 3 tbsp dried)
1 cup vegetable broth
1/2 cup kidney beans (or black eyed peas) cooked
1/3 cup lime juice (or lemon)
Bragg liquid aminos to taste (optional)

Directions

1. Heat oil in non-stick skillet.
2. Sauté onions until translucent.
3. Add seitan and tumeric and sauté till lightly brown.
4. Stir in parsley, leeks, and fenugreek; sauté for 5 minutes.
5. Add broth, beans, and lime juice and bring to a boil.
6. Lower flame and simmer for 10-15 minutes or until greens are tender.
7. Serve over a bed of rice along with Yogurt Cheese & Shallots (p. 118) or Yogurt Cucumber Sauce (p. 115).

Fenugreek warms, tonifies, and aids digestion.

Stuffed Eggplant, Green Pepper, And Tomato

BASED ON A PERSIAN RECIPE, THIS COLORFUL DISH
IS QUITE A CROWD PLEASER.

Ingredients

2 lg eggplants
Sea salt
2 green peppers
1 lg tomato
2 cups rice, cooked
1 cup yellow split peas, cooked
1/2 cup parsley, chopped
4 green onions, chopped
1 tsp cinnamon
1/2 tsp allspice
1 tsp tumeric
1 tbsp low sodium tamari soy sauce
1 tbsp extra virgin olive oil
1 cup vegetable broth

Directions

1. Cut off eggplant tops plus another 1/2" round. Set aside.
2. Peel eggplants in stripes and scoop out pulp with a small spoon.
3. Sprinkle inside of eggplants with sea salt and set upside down in colander.
4. Cut off top of green peppers and tomato and scoop out pulp and seeds.
5. Keep the tops.
6. In large bowl, mix rice, split peas, parsley, green onions, cinnamon, allspice, tumeric, tamari, and 2 tsp olive oil.

7. Rinse eggplant and pat dry.
8. Stuff eggplant with filling and plug top with extra round cut to fit the opening. Secure with toothpicks.
9. Fill green peppers and tomato with filling and secure top with toothpicks.
10. Lightly oil a casserole dish.
11. Brush stuffed eggplant with remaining oil and bake in casserole dish at 350 degrees F for 15-20 minutes, or until brown.
12. Arrange stuffed peppers and tomato in the casserole dish; add broth.
13. Cover and bake at 350 degrees F for 45 minutes or until vegetables are tender.
14. Serve with plain yogurt or Yogurt Sauce (p. 115) and fresh whole wheat pita or tortilla bread. Serves six - eight.

Allspice helps ease flatulence.

Spinach Prune Stew

A SURPRISINGLY DELICIOUS NEW TASTE SENSATION.

Ingredients

1 onion, chopped
1 tbsp sesame oil
1 tsp tumeric
1/2 lb prunes, pitted (about 25 prunes)
1 tbsp lime juice (or lemon)
2 cups vegetable broth
1 lb spinach, finely chopped

Directions

1. Sauté onion in sesame oil till translucent.
2. Stir in prunes, lime juice, and vegetable broth.
3. Bring to a boil; lower flame and simmer for 20 minutes or until prunes are cooked.
4. Add spinach and simmer for another 5-10 minutes.
5. Serve over a bed of rice, millet, or couscous.
6. Serves four.

Carrot Pilaf

COLORFUL AND TASTY, YET VERY SIMPLE TO MAKE.

Ingredients

1 onion, chopped
1 tbsp sesame oil
4 carrots, cut in match sticks
1/3 cup currants
1/3 cup almonds, slivered
1 1/2 cups brown or basmati rice
2 cups vegetable broth
Bragg liquid aminos to taste (optional)

Directions

1. Sauté onion in sesame oil till translucent.
2. Add carrots, currants, and almonds; sauté for another 5 minutes.
3. In non-stick pot, bring rice and broth to a boil.
4. Stir in carrot mixture and reduce flame to low.
5. Cover lid with towel and simmer for 30-45 minutes.
6. Serve with a fresh green salad.
7. Serves four.

Korean Mung Bean Pancakes

CONTRIBUTED BY CHUNG JA PARK

Ingredients

1 cup mung beans, soaked overnight
2 cups cabbage, finely grated or chopped
2 carrots, coarsely grated
2 cups mung bean sprouts
1 bunch green onions, cut in threes and sliced lengthwise
1 tsp sea salt (optional)
2 cloves garlic, minced
1/2 tsp fresh ginger, minced
Sesame oil

Sauce

2 tbsp low sodium tamari soy sauce
2 tbsp rice vinegar
2 tbsp water

Directions

Toss vegetables with salt and let sit for 10 minutes.
Drain beans and grind finely in blender or food processor.
Squeeze out excess water from vegetables.
Mix with bean paste, garlic, and ginger.
Heat oil and drop mixture by large spoonfuls. Flatten out with spatula.
Brown on both sides and serve with dipping sauce, cooked grain (rice, millet, or buckwheat), and green salad.
Serves four - six.

Mung beans are cleansing and easy to digest

Chinese Stir Fry

A Very Healthy Dish With A Minimum Of Prep Time.

Ingredients

1 tbsp sesame oil
3 cloves garlic, minced
1 tsp fresh ginger, grated
1/2 lb tofu, cubed
2 carrots, cut diagonally and thinly
1 cup bok choy, chopped
1 cup broccoli florettes
1 red bell pepper, cut in strips

Sauce

1 tbsp low sodium Tamari soy sauce
1 tbsp maple syrup or honey
1 tbsp kuzu (or arrowroot powder)
1/2 cup water
1/4 cup sherry (optional)

Directions

Mix sauce ingredients in a blender and set aside.
Heat sesame oil in wok until it sizzles.
Add garlic and ginger and cook for one minute, stirring constantly.
Stir in tofu and fry for 3 minutes, over medium-high flame, until lightly brown.
Add remaining vegetables and stir fry for 3-5 minutes or until vegetables are cooked al dente (lightly cooked, but firm).
Pour in sauce and mix well until sauce thickens, 1-3 minutes.
Serve over a bed of rice.
Serves four - six.

Spinach & Eggs

A QUICK, SIMPLE WAY TO GET YOUR PROTEIN AND GREENS.

Ingredients

4 cups spinach, chopped
1 onion, chopped
1 tbsp extra virgin olive oil
6 egg whites or 3 eggs, beaten
1 tsp kelp granules or powder

Directions

1. Steam spinach for 5-8 minutes.
2. Sauté onion in olive oil until golden.
3. Mix in spinach and cook for 1 minute.
4. Add eggs and kelp. Cook over low flame until eggs are set.
5. Serve with whole wheat pita or tortilla bread.

Swedish Wheatballs

NO ONE WILL MISS THE MEAT IN THIS TASTY ADAPTATION OF A POPULAR DISH FROM SWEDEN.

Ingredients

1 cup TVP (texturized vegetable protein)
2 tbsp vegetarian bacon bits
2/3 cup vegetable broth, hot
1 cup whole wheat bread crumbs
2 egg whites or 1 egg, beaten
1/2 tsp Worcestershire sauce (vegetarian preferred)
1/2 tsp allspice, ground

Gravy

1 cup vegetable broth
1-2 tbsp kuzu or arrowroot powder
1-2 tbsp water

Directions

1. In medium bowl, mix TVP, bacon bits, and hot broth.
2. Cover and let sit for 10 minutes.
3. Mix all ingredients and form into 1 1/2 inch balls.
4. Place in non-stick or lightly oiled baking dish and bake at 400 degrees F for 25 minutes or until lightly brown.
5. Heat vegetable broth.
6. Dissolve kuzu in water and add to broth.
7. Simmer, stirring constantly, until gravy thickens.

8. Serve over wheatballs along with a cooked grain and fresh green salad.
9. Serves four - six.

Suggestion:

If wheatball mixture is too moist, add 1-2 tbsp whole wheat flour.

Tofu Tacos

A ZESTY TREAT FROM MEXICO.

Ingredients

1 lg onion, chopped
2 cloves garlic, minced
2 tbsp sesame oil
1 lb tofu, previously frozen and thawed
2 tsp cumin powder
1 tbsp Bragg liquid aminos
6-8 taco shells (or corn tortillas)
1 1/2 cup lettuce mixed with other greens of your choice
1 lg tomato, chopped
Mild taco sauce
1/2 cup feta cheese, crumbled, or soy cheese, shredded (optional)

Directions

1. Sauté onion and garlic in sesame oil til golden.
2. Squeeze excess water out of tofu and pat dry.
3. Shred tofu and mix in with onion and garlic.
4. Add cumin and Bragg liquid aminos; brown lightly.
5. Serve tofu mixture in taco shells or heated tortillas folded over.
6. Top with lettuce and greens, tomatoes, sauce, and cheese.
7. Serves four - six.

Corn tortillas are a source of calcium.

Fettuccini Light

ENJOY THIS DELIGHTFUL DISH WITHOUT HAVING TO WORRY ABOUT THE FAT!

Ingredients

1 tbsp extra virgin olive oil
2 cloves garlic, minced
1 1/2 cups rice milk
3 tbsp wheat flour
1/3 cup brewer's yeast
1 pkg whole wheat fettuccine
1 tbsp Bragg liquid aminos or low sodium tamari soy sauce
1 cup broccoli florrettes
2 carrots, sliced diagonally
1 cup Chinese pea pods
Fresh basil for garnish

Directions

1. Sauté garlic in olive oil until lightly brown.
2. Add flour and make a roux.
3. Slowly add rice milk, mixing briskly to avoid lumping.
4. Let mixture simmer, stirring frequently, until sauce thickens.
5. Stir in brewers yeast and whisk to avoid lumpiness.
6. Set aside.
7. Cook pasta according to package directions. Drain and rinse.
8. Return to pot and toss with Bragg or soy sauce.
9. Steam vegetables for 10 minutes or until cooked al dente.
10. Serve vegetables spread over a bed of pasta, topped with sauce.
11. Garnish with basil.
12. Serves four.

Burdock Burgers

HEALTHY COMPETITION FOR THE FAMOUS GARDEN BURGER.

Ingredients

1/2 lb tofu, drained
1 small carrot, grated
1 medium burdock root, grated
1/2 small onion, grated
4 mushrooms, finely chopped
2 tbsp miso paste
1/3 cup brewer's yeast
1/4 cup wheat germ (MUST be fresh)
1 tbsp sesame oil
1/4 cup whole wheat bread crumbs

Directions

1. Slice tofu and wrap in several layers of paper towel; press to remove excess moisture.
2. Crumble tofu and add carrot, burdock, onion, mushrooms, miso, brewer's yeast, and wheat germ; mix well.
3. Form mixture into four patties. (If too moist, add more brewer's yeast or wheat germ).
4. Coat patties with bread crumbs and brown on lightly oiled griddle or bake on lightly oiled baking sheet at 350 degrees F for 10-15 minutes or until golden.
5. Flip patties to brown on both side.

6. Serve with steamed veggies and potatoes or grain, or enjoy as a hot sandwich with whole grain toast, lettuce, and tomato.
7. Serves four.

Burdock is a potent blood cleanser.

Egyptian Bean Medley

AN ORIGINAL DISH FROM THE LAND OF THE NILE.
CONTRIBUTED BY NONNA SEIFALLA

Ingredients

1 cup fava beans, dried (smaller beans preferred)
5 cups water (x3)
2 cloves garlic, crushed
1/2 green pepper, chopped
1/2 yellow pepper, chopped
1/2 red pepper, chopped
1 tomato, chopped
4 green onions, chopped
1/2 cup parsley, chopped
1/2 cup dill weed, chopped (or 1/2 tbsp dried)
2 tbsp sesame tahini
2 tsp cumin, ground
1 tsp paprika, ground (optional)
2 tsp Bragg liquid aminos (optional)

Directions

1. Bring beans and water to a boil; drain.
2. Repeat above procedure.
3. Add beans to last five cups of water and bring to a boil.
4. Lower flame and simmer until tender, about one hour.
5. Add additional water if necessary.
6. When beans are well-cooked, and liquid is reduced to about 1 1/2 cups, add garlic, cumin, and paprika.
7. Cook for 2-3 minutes.
8. Stir in tahini. If too thick, add a little water.

9. Add tomatoes, peppers, and green onions.
10. Cook for another 2-3 minutes, stirring occasionally. (Beans will have fallen apart and mixture will look like a paste)
11. Stir in parsley and dill. Season with Bragg liquid aminos and serve with warm pitta bread.
12. Serves four - six.

Suggestion

Break 3-4 eggs on top of mixture. Cover, and cook over low flame until eggs are set. Eggs may also be mixed in.

If beans are large and have an outer skin, you may need to peel them after the first boiling as the skins will be too tough. Some Middle Eastern food stores will carry small or peeled beans.

Sweet peppers are a good source of vitamin C.

Green Bean Pilaf

THE COMBINATION OF CUMIN AND CINNAMON GIVE THIS DISH A FLAVOR ALL ITS OWN.

Ingredients

1 1/2 cup brown or basmati rice
3 cups vegetable broth
1/2 lb green beans, cut in 1/2 inch pieces and steamed al dente
2 ripe tomatoes, chopped (or 2 tbsp tomato paste)
1 tbsp cumin seeds
1 tsp cinnamon

Directions

1. In medium, non-stick pot, bring rice, broth, beans, and tomatoes to a boil.
2. Reduce heat to low.
3. Toast cumin seeds in non-stick skillet.
4. Add to rice along with cinnamon.
5. Wrap lid in towel and simmer for 35-45 minutes.
6. Serve with Yogurt Sauce (p. 115), Yogurt Cheese with Shallots (p. 118), or a fresh green salad.
7. Serve four.

Suggestions

For added protein, sauté 1/2 lb cubed tofu and one chopped onion in 1 tbsp sesame oil. Season with Bragg liquid aminos and serve with rice.

Sausage & Sauerkraut

A SWISS FAVORITE FOR COLD WINTER NIGHTS.
ADAPTED FROM A RECIPE CONTRIBUTED BY HEIDI TSCHANZ

Ingredients

3-4 potatoes, quartered
1 onion, chopped
1 tbsp canola oil
8 meatless sausage, sliced
2 tsp caraway seeds
1 cup vegetable broth
1 apple, peeled and grated
1 tsp apple cider vinegar
1 cup sauerkraut
Plain, nonfat yogurt (optional)

Directions

1. Steam potatoes till tender.
2. Heat oil and sauté onion and sausage till brown.
3. Add caraway seeds and cook for 1-2 minutes.
4. Include broth, apple, and apple cider vinegar.
5. Bring to a boil.
6. Lower flame and stir in sauerkraut.
7. Simmer 1-2 minutes to blend flavors. Do not boil.
8. Serve topped with a dollop of yogurt and potatoes on the side with whole grain bread.
9. Serves four.

Caraway seeds increase breast milk and freshen breath.

Nutloaf With Mushroom Gravy

NO MEATLOAF HAS THE EDGE ON THIS VEGETARIAN VERSIAN.

Ingredients

1 lb tofu, drained
1 cup scotch mix (mixed rolled grains), or rolled oats
1/2 cup vegetable broth, hot
1/4 cup whole wheat flour or wheat germ
3 tbsp miso paste
1 cup walnuts, finely chopped
1/4 cup parsley, chopped
1 small onion, grated
2 egg whites or 1 egg (optional, but helps loaf hold its shape)
1 tsp sesame oil

Gravy

6 mushrooms, sliced
1 tbsp sesame oil
1 cup vegetable broth
1 tbsp kuzu or arrowroot
1 tsp low sodium Tamari soy sauce

Directions

1. Slice tofu and wrap in paper towel.
2. Press to release excess moisture.
3. Crumble into a bowl.
4. Moisten rolled grains with hot broth.
5. Mix in with tofu along with other ingredients except oil and mix well.
6. Lightly oil loaf pan and press in mixture.

7. Bake at 350 degrees F for 30 minutes.
8. Sauté mushrooms in oil till tender.
9. Blend vegetable broth, kuzu, and soy sauce.
10. Add to mushrooms and simmer until sauce thickens, about 5 minutes.
11. Remove loaf from pan and top with gravy.
12. Serve with steamed veggies and potatoes.
13. Serves six - eight.

Suggestions

Leftovers make great sandwiches, hot or cold.

Green Beans & Eggs

SIMPLY DELICIOUS AND GREAT FOR A POTLUCK.

Ingredients

1 lb fresh green beans
1 onion, chopped
1 tbsp extra virgin olive oil
6 egg whites, beaten (or 3 eggs)
Bragg liquid aminos to taste

Directions

1. Cut beans in threes and steam for 8-10 minutes or until tender.
2. Sauté onion in olive oil til golden.
3. Add green beans to onion mixture and cook, stirring frequently, for one minute.
4. Stir in eggs and mix well.
5. Cook for 1-2 minutes, or until eggs are set.
6. Season with Bragg liquid aminos and serve with whole grain bread.
7. Serves four.

Broccoli Cauliflower Casserole

THE CANCER-PREVENTING BENEFIT OF TWO VEGETABLES IN ONE SIMPLE DISH.

Ingredients

1 1/2 lb broccoli florets
1 1/2 lb cauliflower florets
1 1/2 tbsp canola oil
4 tbsp unbleached flour
2 cups soy milk
1 tsp onion powder
1/4 tsp nutmeg
1/3 cup sherry
1 bay leaf
1/2 tsp sea salt (optional)
Dash of cayenne (optional)
2-3 oz feta cheese, rinsed and crumbled

Directions

1. Steam broccoli and cauliflower florets for 5-7 minutes.
2. Heat oil and add flour to make a roux.
3. Slowly add soy milk, stirring briskly to avoid lumping.
4. Add onion powder, nutmeg, sherry, bay leaf, sea salt, and cayenne.
5. Simmer for 5-8 minutes, stirring regularly, until sauce thickens.
6. Arrange broccoli and cauliflower florets in 9x13 casserole dish.
7. Pour sauce over vegetables and sprinkle with Feta cheese.
8. Bake at 350 degrees F for 25-30 minutes.
9. Serve with cooked grain or whole grain bread.
10. Serves four - six.

Broccoli is a source of calcium and vitamin C.

Rice & Black-Eyed Peas

A COMPLETE PROTEIN ALL IN ONE POT.

Ingredients

1 1/2 cups brown or basmati rice
1 cup black-eyed peas, cooked
1/2 cup fresh dill weed, chopped
1 tsp sea salt (optional)
Bragg liquid aminos to taste

Directions

1. Wash rice and put in non-stick pot along with black-eyed peas, dill weed, and sea salt.
2. Bring to a boil.
3. Reduce heat and wrap lid with towel.
4. Simmer 35-45 minutes over low flame.
5. Serve with plain yogurt.
6. Serves four.

Stuffed Spinach Mushroom Loaf

GOOD HOT OR COLD, A FRESH NEW WAY TO EAT YOUR GREENS.

Ingredients

1 onion, chopped
1 tbsp extra virgin olive oil
1/2 lb mushrooms, sliced
2 cups spinach, finely chopped
2 cups collard greens, finely chopped
Dough for one loaf whole wheat bread
3-4 oz feta cheese, rinsed and crumbled

Directions

1. Sauté onion in olive oil til translucent.
2. Add mushrooms and cook till tender.
3. Mix in spinach and collard.
4. Cook over low flame for 5-7 minutes or until tender and liquid is totally absorbed.
5. Roll out bread dough and spread mixture.
6. Sprinkle with feta cheese and roll into the shape of a loaf.
7. Fold over and secure ends to keep filling inside.
8. Bake in conventional oven according to dough directions.
9. Let cool for 15 minutes.
10. Slice and serve with fresh green salad.
11. Serves four - six.

Potato Tomato Rice

SERVE WITH SAUTÉED SEITAN OR TOFU FOR A COMPLETE MEAL.

Ingredients

1 1/2 cups brown or basmati rice
3 cups vegetable broth
2 tomatoes, chopped
2 potatoes, cut into bite-size cubes
1 green pepper, chopped
1 tsp sea salt (optional)
1 tsp cinnamon
1 tbsp cumin seeds

Directions

1. Wash rice. In non-stick pot, bring rice and broth to a boil.
2. Mix in tomatoes, potatoes, green pepper, and sea salt.
3. Toast cumin seeds in non-stick pan or toaster oven.
4. Add cinnamon and cumin seeds to rice.
5. Wrap lid in towel and simmer over low flame for 35-45 minutes.
6. Serve with fresh green salad.
7. Serves four.

Cinnamon helps improve circulation.

Steamed Veggie Basket

A SIMPLE, YET COLORFUL DISH FOR A SNACK OR LIGHT MEAL

Ingredients

Choose four or more of the following vegetables:
- Potatoes, thinly sliced
- Sweet potatoes, thinly sliced
- Chinese pea pods
- Carrots, thinly sliced
- Asparagus spears
- Broccoli florets
- Cauliflower florets
- Mushrooms
- Green beans
- Zucchini
- Yellow summer squash
- Tofu, cut in bite-size cubes

Sauce

Choose from any of the following sauces, dips, or dressings, or try two or more for variety.
- Tofu Garlic Herb Dip (p. 125)
- Miso Dressing (p. 127)
- Yogurt Herb Dressing (p. 128)
- Avocado Dressing (p. 131)
- Tahina (p. 119)
- Garbanzo Spread (p. 121)
- Tofu Almond Spread (p. 123)

Directions

1. Arrange vegetables in sections in two tiered steaming basket. (If you do not have a steaming basket, steam in something else and arrange on a platter)
2. Place harder vegetables such as potatoes or carrots together.
3. Steam for 10 minutes.
4. Place other vegetables in second tier and put on top of first tier.
5. Steam both tiers together for 10 minutes or until vegetables are cooked, but firm.
6. Serve vegetables in steaming baskets with dipping sauce on the side.

Asparagus is a potent diuretic.

Pizza Verde

IF YOU'RE A PIZZA LOVER, YOU WILL SURELY ENJOY THESE HEALTHY ALTERNATIVES.

Ingredients

1 medium whole grain pizza crust
1 tbsp extra virgin olive oil
4 cups greens (spinach, collard, chard, or a combination), chopped
1 tsp rosemary
1 cup crumbled feta cheese

Directions

1. Brush pizza crust with olive oil and set aside.
2. Wash greens and wilt in non- stick pan, about 2-3 minutes.
3. Remove all moisture and spread over pizza crust.
4. Sprinkle with rosemary and cheese.
5. Bake at 450 degrees F for 10 minutes or until crust is golden.
6. Serves four.

Suggestions

Replace greens with sliced zucchini and yellow summer squash; sprinkle with fresh or dried oregano and feta cheese.

Replace greens with slices of red, yellow, and green peppers. Sprinkle with feta cheese. After baking, garnish with fresh basil leaves.

SAUCES, SNACKS, AND SIDE DISHES

Sweet Potato Bake

THE DISTINCTION BETWEEN DINNER AND DESSERT FADE WITH THIS NUTRITIOUS SIDE DISH.

Ingredients

4 sweet potatoes or yams, cooked and mashed
6 egg whites (or 3 eggs), lightly beaten
1/2 tsp cardomon
2 tsp sesame or canola oil
1/4 cup almonds, sliced

Directions

1. Mix potatoes, eggs, and cardomon.
2. Oil pie dish with one teaspoon oil.
3. Pour in egg and potato mixture and spread evenly.
4. Sprinkle almonds over top and drizzle with remaining oil.
5. Bake at 350 degrees F for 15-20 minutes or until set.
6. Serves four - six.

Sweet potatoes are rich in beta carotene and minerals.

Root Roast

ROASTED WITH AROMATIC HERBS, ROOT VEGETABLES MAKE A SPLENDID ACCOMPANIMENT TO ANY MEAL.

Ingredients

Choose one or more of the following roots:
Potatoes, cubed (use alone, or add later, as they tend to cook faster than some of the hardier roots such as rutabaga and beets).
Rutabagas, cubed
Turnips, cubed
Beets, cubed
Kohlrabi, cubed
Carrots, cut in 1 inch pieces
1 tsp sage
1 tsp marjoram
1 tsp thyme
1 tbsp extra virgin olive oil

Directions

1. Toss root vegetables with herbs and olive oil.
2. Put in separate sections in a shallow baking dish.
3. Cover and bake at 350 degrees F for 45 minutes or until vegetables are tender.
4. Check occasionally and stir to avoid sticking.

Nishimi Vegetables

THIS JAPANESE METHOD OF COOKING BRINGS OUT
THE NATURAL SWEETNESS OF THE ROOTS..

Ingredients

1 pc kombu seaweed
2-3 carrots
2 turnips
1 daikon root
1 1/2 cups water
1 tbsp tamari soy sauce

Directions

1. Soak kombu seaweed in cold water for 10 minutes.
2. Drain and cut into small squares.
3. Peel and cut carrots, turnips, and daikon root, all the same bite-size pieces.
4. Place kombu in the bottom of a pot.
5. Top with vegetables, each in a separate section.
6. Add water and bring to a boil.
7. Cover and simmer over low flame for 25-35 minutes.
8. Add tamari and mix.
9. Cook another 5-10 minutes, or until all liquid has been absorbed.

Daikon helps dissolve fat.

Stuffed Potatoes

SERVED WITH A FRESH SALAD, THIS CAN BE A MEAL IN ITSELF.

Ingredients

4 lg potatoes, baked
1 onion, chopped
1/2 lb mushrooms, sliced
1 tbsp extra virgin olive oil
3-4 tbsp pumpkin or sunflower seeds, lightly toasted
1/2 tsp kelp granules or powder
1/2 tsp thyme, dried

Directions

1. Cut a thin layer off the top of each potato.
2. Scoop out middle into a medium bowl.
3. Sauté' onion and mushrooms in olive oil till tender.
4. Mix onion and mushrooms with potato insides.
5. Fold in pumpkin seeds and season with kelp and thyme.
6. Scoop mixture back into potatoes.
7. Brush top of potatoes with olive oil.
8. Place potatoes under broiler for 5 minutes or until brown on top.
9. Serves four.

Pumpkin seeds are a good source of zinc.

Rice Balls

A SIMPLE SNACK, HIGH IN NUTRITION AND LOW IN CALORIES.
ADAPTED FROM A RECIPE CONTRIBUTED BY YOSHI YAMADA

Ingredients

2 cups brown or Japanese rice, well-cooked
1 tbsp rice vinegar
2 tbsp toasted sesame seeds

Filling (Choose One From The Following)

4 umeboshi plums (prepared sour plums)
1/2 cucumber, chopped
2 eggs, cooked and chopped
1 carrot, grated

Dipping Sauce

1 tbsp low sodium tamari soy sauce
1 tbsp rice vinegar
2 tbsp water

Directions

1. Mix rice with vinegar.
2. In shallow cup, place a 12x12 piece of plastic food wrap with the extra parts hanging over the side..
3. Sprinkle 1 tsp sesame seeds into the cup and top with 1/4 cup rice.
4. Press rice firmly into cup.
5. Add the filling and top with 1/4 cup of rice.
6. Press firmly and pull rice ball out of cup, wrapping with plastic.
7. Mold with hands to assure it sticks together.

8. Repeat procedure for 3 additional rice balls.
9. Mix sauce ingredients and serve with rice balls.

Suggestions

Use nori seaweed strips or flakes instead of sesame seeds.

If using brown rice, it must be very soft; otherwise, the rice ball will fall apart.

Umeboshi plums aid digestion and help keep the blood alkaline.

Tofu Sushi

FISH IS NOT THE ONLY THING THAT CAN GO INTO A SUSHI. THIS VERSION WAS SERVED AT MY WEDDING, AND I HAD BARELY TASTED ONE BEFORE THEY ALL DISAPPEARED!

Ingredients

1/4 lb tofu, drained and pat dry
1 carrot, grated
1 rib celery, finely chopped
2 green onions, finely chopped
1 tsp ginger root, grated (or dry powder)
1 tbsp low sodium tamari soy sauce
1 1/2 tbsp soy mayonnaise
1 sm cucumber, cut into thin sticks
1 1/2 cups brown or Japanese rice, well-cooked
3-4 sheets nori seaweed

Directions

1. In medium bowl, crumble tofu and mix with carrot, celery, green onion, ginger, soy sauce, and mayonnaise.
2. Toast nori sheets over medium flame for 3-4 seconds.
3. Place on 12x12 piece of plastic wrap (or sushi mat if you have one)
4. Spread cooked rice about 1/2 inch deep over nori sheet, leaving 1 ½ inches empty at the top and 1/2 inch along the other three sides.
5. Press rice down so that it sticks together.
6. At the bottom of the rice, spread a thin line of tofu mixture and a single line of cucumber sticks.
7. Slowly roll sushi, using plastic wrap and pressing down firmly.
8. Push in sides so mixture doesn't fall out.

9. Remove excess rice and slightly moisten the top of the nori seaweed for it to stick.
10. Wrap nori in plastic wrap and chill.
11. With a sharp knife, cut in 1/2 inch circles and serve with a side of soy sauce as a dip.
12. Makes about 36 rounds.

Suggestions

Cut sushi in half instead of rounds and take it to work for lunch.

Use 1/2 brown rice and 1/2 Japanese or Jasmine rice to help sushi stick together better.

Brown rice is an excellent source of fiber, complex carbohydrates, vitamins, and minerals.

Sautéed Greens

A QUICK MINERAL-RICH ADDITION TO ANY MEAL.

Ingredients

2 cloves garlic, chopped
1 onion, chopped
1 tbsp sesame oil
4 cups greens, chopped (spinach, kale, collard, chard, or amaranth)
1/2 cup vegetable broth
Dash of sherry (optional)
Bragg liquid aminos

Directions

1. Sauté garlic and onion in sesame oil til brown.
2. Add vegetable broth and bring to a boil.
3. Lower heat and mix in greens.
4. Season with sherry and Bragg (alcohol will evaporate)
5. Simmer for 5-8 minutes or until greens are tender and liquid is absorbed.

Dark leafy green vegetables contain disease fighting phytochemicals.

Fresh Herb Roll-Up

AN AROMATIC SNACK; FRESH FROM THE GARDEN.

Ingredients

Whole wheat flat bread (Lahvosh, tortilla, or chapati)
Yogurt Cheese (yogurt strained through a cloth overnight in the refrigerator) or feta cheese
Green onions, sliced lengthwise
Fresh basil leaves
Fresh tarragon leaves

Directions

1. Spread pieces of flat bread with cheese.
2. Top with fresh herbs.
3. Roll up and serve as a snack or light lunch.

Suggestions

Replace herbs with sliced cucumber and tomatoes.

Yogurt-Cucumber Sauce

SIMPLE AND CALCIUM RICH, USE AS A SAUCE, DIP, OR SIDE DISH.

Ingredients

32 oz. plain non-fat yogurt
1 cucumber, finely chopped
2 green onions, chopped
1 tsp dried mint
1 tbsp fresh dill weed, chopped (or 1 tsp dried)
Sea salt to taste (optional)

Directions

1. Mix all ingredients and chill.

Suggestions

Serve with rice dishes, tortilla chips, raw vegetables, or pita bread.

Yogurt supplies the colon with beneficial bacteria.

Spinach & Yogurt

A Low-Cal Nutritious Dip, Sauce, Or Side Dish.

Ingredients

1 bunch fresh spinach
1 cup nonfat plain yogurt
1-2 tsp garlic powder
1 tsp kelp granules or powder (or 1/2 tsp sea salt)

Directions

1. Steam spinach for 5-8 minutes or until tender.
2. Squeeze out excess water and finely chop.
3. Mix yogurt, spinach, garlic powder, and kelp.
4. Chill and serve with whole wheat pita wedges, whole wheat crackers, or nonfat tortilla chips.

Beets & Yogurt

A FRESH NEW WAY TO SERVE BEETS.

Ingredients

3-4 beets, peeled and cut into bite-size pieces
2 cups nonfat plain yogurt

Directions

1. Steam beets for 15-20 minutes or until tender.
2. Fold into yogurt and chill.
3. Serve as a side dish.

Beets help cleanse the blood.

Yogurt Cheese With Shallots

A Tasty Accompaniment To Any Rice Dish.

Ingredients

2 cups nonfat plain yogurt
5-6 shallots, chopped
1/2 tsp sea salt (optional)

Directions

1. Strain yogurt in cheese cloth hanging over a bowl (in refrigerator) over night.
2. Peel shallots and soak in water overnight.
3. Chop or thinly slice shallots and fold into yogurt cheese.
4. Season with salt and chill for flavors to mix.
5. Serve with rice dish, especially Lima-Dill Pilaf (p. 41) and Herbed Rice (p. 70).

Tahina

A CALCIUM-RICH MIDDLE EASTERN DIP.
CONTRIBUTED BY *NONNA SEIFALLA*

Ingredients

1 cup sesame tahini, roasted
4-5 cloves garlic, crushed
3 tbsp lemon or lime juice
3 tbsp apple cider vinegar
1 tbsp + 1 tsp cumin powder
2/3 cup water

Directions

1. Mix all ingredients in blender until smooth.
2. Dip should look almost white.
3. Chill and serve with pita wedges, whole grain crackers, fresh or lightly steamed vegetables.

Suggestions

Adjust water to desired consistency.
Garnish with parsley leaves and sliced black olives.

Sesame seeds are an excellent source of protein and calcium.

Lentil Pate'

**PROTEIN RICH AND PREPARED IN MINUTES.
DELICIOUS IN ITS SIMPLICITY.**

Ingredients

1 cup brown lentils, well-cooked
1 tsp oregano
1 tsp sea salt (optional)
1 tbsp extra virgin olive oil

Directions

1. Mash lentils well.
2. Mix in oregano, sea salt, and olive oil.
3. Serve with pita wedges or whole grain crackers.

Suggestions

Wrap up leftovers in a whole wheat tortilla along with green onions and fresh basil for a light lunch or snack.

Garbanzo Spread

MIXED WITH AROMATIC INDIAN SPICES, THIS SPREAD IS AN EXOTIC TREAT.

Ingredients

1 1/2 cup garbanzo beans, cooked
1 tsp cumin powder
1/2 tsp coriander powder
1/2 tsp tumeric
1/4 tsp ginger
Dash of cayenne (optional)
2 tsp Bragg liquid aminos
1 tbsp extra virgin olive oil
1/4 cup water

Directions

1. Blend all ingredients and chill.
2. Serve with nonfat tortillas, pita wedges, or fresh vegetables.

Suggestions

Also great wrapped up with veggies in a whole wheat tortilla.

Coriander aids digestion.

Fava Bean Dip

A Protein-Rich Dip From The Middle East.
Contributed By *Nonna Seifalla*

Ingredients

1 cup fava beans, dried (smaller beans preferred)
4 cups water (x3)
1 tbsp cumin powder
1 tsp garlic powder
1 tbsp extra virgin olive oil
1-2 lemons, juiced

Directions

1. Bring beans to a boil in 4 cups water.
2. Drain and repeat procedure.
3. Return beans to pot along with final 4 cups of water and simmer, over low flame for 45 minutes to 1 hour, or until beans are tender.
4. Drain water and mash beans.
5. Mix in cumin, garlic, olive oil, and juice of one lemon.
6. Slice remaining lemon in wedges and serve on the side.
7. Add extra lemon according to personal taste.
8. Serve with whole wheat pita bread and a fresh green salad.

Suggestions

If beans are too large, the outer skin will be tough. In this case, it is better to peel off the outer skins after the first boil. They come off easily.

Tofu Almond Spread

RICH IN PROTEIN AND CALCIUM.

Ingredients

1/2 lb tofu, drained
1/2 cup almond butter
1 tbsp flax seeds
1 tbsp sesame oil
3 lemons, juiced
2 tbsp plain, nonfat yogurt
Pinch of sea salt (optional)

Directions

1. Blend all ingredients till smooth.
2. Serve with whole grain crackers, fresh or steamed vegetables, or use as a sauce with cooked vegetables.

Flax seeds are an excellent source of essential fatty acids.

Homemade Seitan (Wheat Gluten)

THERE ARE A VARIETY OF WAYS TO MAKE SEITAN.
THIS IN MY VERSION.

Ingredients

1 cup wheat gluten (available in natural food stores as flour)
1/2 cup water
1/3 cup low sodium tamari soy sauce
2 quarts water
1 pc kombu seaweed
1/3 cup low sodium tamari soy sauce

Directions

1. In large bowl, mix gluten, water, and 1/3 cup soy sauce.
2. Knead for a few minutes until you have a smooth ball.
3. Bring water, kombu seaweed, and soy sauce to a boil.
4. Place gluten ball in water and lower heat.
5. Simmer for 2 hours.
6. Drain and slice or cube and use in your favorite dish.
7. This will keep up to one week in the refrigerator.
8. Makes about 1 lb seitan.

Seitan is high protein, low fat, and cholesterol free.

Tofu Garlic Herb Dip

Ingredients

1/2 lb tofu, drained
2 tsp garlic powder
3 tbsp lemon juice
2 tbsp light miso
2 tsp extra virgin olive oil
2/3 cup water
2 tbsp fresh parsley, chopped
2 tbsp fresh chives, chopped

Directions

1. Blend tofu, garlic powder, lemon juice, miso, olive oil, and water till smooth.
2. Fold in parsley and chives and serve with fresh veggies.

Suggestion

Add more water and serve as a salad dressing.

Parsley is beneficial to the eyes, kidney, and liver.

Oriental Dressing

ADD AN EXOTIC FLAVOR TO ANY SALAD WITH THIS JAPANESE DRESSING.

Ingredients

2 tbsp sesame oil, roasted
1 1/2 tbsp low sodium tamari soy sauce
1 1/2 tbsp rice vinegar
2 tbsp mirin (or honey or maple syrup)
1/4 cup water
1 tbsp sesame seeds, roasted

Directions

1. Mix all ingredients and serve over your favorite salad.

Suggestions

Add small amount of water if flavor is too strong.

Miso Dressing

ENJOY THE MANY BENEFITS OF MISO IN THIS DELIGHTFUL DRESSING.

Ingredients

3 tbsp light miso paste
1/4 cup sesame tahini
2 garlic cloves, crushed
1 1/2 tbsp maple syrup
1 1/2 tbsp rice vinegar
1/3 cup water

Directions

1. Blend all ingredients and serve.

Suggestion

For added zest, mix in 1 tsp chili powder and 1 tsp Italian herbs.

Garlic is a source of selenium, an anti-cancer agent.

Yogurt Herb Dressing

Light, And Simple To Make, This Dressing Is A Winner.

Ingredients

1 cup plain non-fat yogurt
3 tbsp fresh dill, chopped (or 2 tsp dried)
2 tbsp soy mayonnaise
1/2 tsp kelp powder
2 green onions, finely chopped
1 tsp garlic powder
1 tsp Bragg liquid aminos
Dash of cayenne

Directions

1. Mix all ingredients and serve over your favorite salad.

Dill increases mother's milk.

Lemon Dressing

DELICIOUS IN ITS SIMPLICITY, ENJOY THIS MIDDLE EASTERN FAVORITE ON ANY VEGETABLE SALAD.

Ingredients

1/4 cup lemon or lime juice, freshly squeezed
2-3 tbsp extra virgin olive oil
2 tbsp parley, finely chopped
1 tsp Bragg liquid aminos

Directions

1. Mix all ingredients and serve.

Herb Vinegar Dressing

THE SAVORY HERBS ADD A SPECIAL FLAVOR TO THIS VINEGARETTE.

Ingredients

1/4 cup wine vinegar
2-3 tbsp extra virgin olive oil
1/2 tsp tarragon
1/2 tsp thyme
1/2 tsp rosemary

Directions

1. Mix all ingredients and serve.

Suggestions

If taste of vinegar is too sharp, mix with a little water before adding olive oil and herbs.

Tarragon helps promote menses.

Avocado Dressing

A SMOOTH, CREAMY DRESSING.

Ingredients

1 avocado, mashed
1 clove garlic, crushed
1/4 cup fresh basil, chopped
2-3 tbsp lemon juice
1 tbsp Bragg liquid aminos
1 tbsp soy mayonnaise
1/4 cup water

Directions

1. Mix all ingredients in blender til smooth.
2. If dressing is too thick, add water to desired consistency.
3. Serve with greens.

Avocados are a source of manganese, a nutrient that helps regulate blood sugar.

Avocado Spread

ENJOY THIS SPREAD IN PITA POCKETS WITH SPROUTS AND TOMATOES.

Ingredients

1 avocado, mashed
1/4 cup cilantro, chopped
1/2 small onion, finely chopped
1 tbsp soy mayonnaise
1 tbsp lime juice
1 tbsp Bragg liquid aminos

Directions

1. Mix all ingredients and serve with pita wedges or veggies.

Tofu Vanilla Sauce

A VERSATILE SAUCE TO USE WITH ANY DESSERT.

Ingredients

1/2 lb tofu
1 tsp vanilla
1-2 tbsp lemon juice
1/4 cup maple syrup

Directions

1. Blend all ingredients til smooth.
2. Serve with fresh fruit or as a topping for cake or pie.

On The Side

I Keep the Following on Hand to Serve as an Accompaniment to Grain Dishes:

Fresh cucumber, sliced (source of hormones)
Sauerkraut, low-sodium or homemade (lactic acid)
Daikon, grated (burns fat)
Radish
Green onion
Fresh basil (aids digestion)
Fresh cilantro

I Also Use the Following as Healthy Condiments

Kelp granules or powder (rich in minerals)
Roasted sesame seeds and nori seaweed flakes (calcium sources)
Bragg liquid aminos (replaces salt)
Extra virgin olive oil (heart healthy fat)
Flax seed oil (essential fatty acids)
Fresh lemon or lime (sources of vitamin C)

Drinks and Desserts

Cranberry Spritzer

A REFRESHING SODA ALTERNATIVE WITHOUT THE ADDED SUGAR.

Ingredients

1 cup cranberry juice, 100% pure
1 12-oz can frozen apple juice concentrate
3 1/2 - 4 cups sparkling water

Directions

1. Blend cranberry juice and apple juice concentrate.
2. Mix in sparkling water. Chill and serve.

Suggestions

Do not use blender as it creates too much foam.
Try adding a scoop of vanilla Rice Dream frozen dessert for a refreshing break on a hot summer day.

Cranberries help keep a healthy urinary track.

Cranberry Punch

KID AND CROWD PLEASER.

Ingredients

10 oz frozen apple juice concentrate
1 1/2 cups cranberry juice, 100% pure
3 cups pineapple juice

Directions

1. Mix all ingredients. Chill and serve.

Suggestions

Do not use blender. It creates too much foam.
If juice is too sweet, add water to desired sweetness.

Cranberries are known as a kidney cleanser.

Pineapple Spritzer

A REFRESHING ALTERNATIVE TO SUGAR LADEN SODAS.

Ingredients

1 can pineapple juice concentrate (100% pure juice)
3 - 3 1/2 cups sparkling mineral water

Directions

1. Mix (do not blend) all ingredients. Chill and serve.

Suggestions

Try other 100% pure juice concentrates for a variety of fresh, cool drinks.

Pineapple is a source of vitamins A and C.

Lime Cooler

PLEASANTLY SATISFYING ON A HOT SUMMER AFTERNOON.

Ingredients

1 can white grape juice concentrate (100% juice)
3 cups spring or sparkling water
3-4 limes, juiced

Directions

1. Mix all ingredients, chill, and serve.

Suggestion

Do not blend if using sparkling water.
Replace 1/3 of grape juice concentrate with pink grapefruit for a more colorful drink.

Yogurt Cooler

DRINK YOUR CALCIUM AND COOL DOWN, ALL IN ONE SHOT.

Ingredients

1 cup plain, non-fat yogurt
1 1/2 cups sparkling mineral water
1/2 tsp mint, dried
1 tsp kelp powder

Directions

1. Mix all ingredients. Chill and serve.

Suggestions

Do not use blender. It creates too much foam.
Use water in place of sparkling water.

Watermelon Juice

LIGHT, REFRESHING, AND VERY LOW IN CALORIES!

Ingredients

1 ripe watermelon, seedless

Directions

1. Cut watermelon and scoop out pulp.
2. Blend in batches and strain through a mesh colander.
3. Chill and serve.

Suggestions

Add a small amount of maple syrup or other natural sweetener to taste.

Watermelon is very cooling.

Evening Tea

SOOTHING AND RELAXING, THIS TEA ALSO PROVIDES CALCIUM!

Ingredients

1 part chamomile
1 part peppermint
2 parts oatstraw (Not oatmeal)

Directions

1. Bring water to a boil.
2. Add all ingredients, and simmer on low flame for 10 minutes.
3. Turn off stove and let herbs steep another 10 minutes.
4. Strain and serve.

Suggestions

Serve with a twist of lemon and a bit of honey.

Oatstraw is a source of calcium, while peppermint and chamomile are soothing and calming.

Indian Ginger Tea (Chai)

THIS AROMATIC TEA IS GOOD FOR DIGESTION.

Ingredients

1 4-inch piece fresh ginger root
5 cups water
4-6 cardommon pods
2-3 cinnamon sticks
1 tbsp (2 teabags) green or black tea (optional)
Rice or soy milk
Honey or maple syrup to taste (optional)

Directions

1. Cut ginger into small pieces.
2. In large pot, bring ginger, water, cardommon, and cinnamon to a boil.
3. Lower heat and simmer for 20-30 minutes.
4. Turn off stove and add tea.
5. Let steep for 5 minutes.
6. Strain and serve with rice or soy milk.
7. Sweeten with honey or maple syrup.

Suggestions

For an extra creamy tea, try soy malt in place of soy milk.

Green tea balances the PH of the body. A potent source of antioxidants, it may help prevent premature aging and some diseases.

Hibiscus Ginger Ice Tea

DELIGHTFUL AND REFRESHING.

Ingredients

1 4-inch piece fresh ginger
5 cups water
3-4 tbsp hibiscus, dried (or tea bags)
Honey to taste

Directions

1. Cut ginger into small pieces.
2. In large pot, bring ginger and water to a boil.
3. Lower heat and simmer for 30 minutes.
4. Turn off stove and add hibiscus.
5. Steep for 5-8 minutes.
6. Sweeten with honey and chill.

Cantaloupe Smoothie

A SIMPLE WAY TO GET YOUR VITAMINS.

Ingredients

1 ripe cantaloupe
1 cup crushed ice
1/4 tsp nutmeg
Mint leaves for garnish

Directions

1. Cut cantaloupe and scoop out pulp.
2. Blend with other ingredients till smooth.
3. Serve in tall glasses garnished with mint leaves.

Cantaloupe is a source of vitamins A and C.

Banana Yogurt Smoothie

SO NUTRITIOUS, ITS PRACTICALLY A MEAL BY ITSELF.

Ingredients

1 cup plain nonfat yogurt
2 bananas, frozen
1 tbsp bee pollen
1-2 tbsp maple syrup (or to taste)
1 tsp vanilla
1/2 cup water
Nutmeg or cinnamon (optional)

Directions

1. Blend all ingredients til smooth.
2. Serve in tall glasses.
3. Sprinkle with nutmeg or cinnamon.

Bee pollen is antimierobial. It is also a rich source of B vitamins, enzymes, amino acids, and minerals.

Hawaiian Sorbet

YOU DON'T HAVE TO MISS YOUR DESSERT THIS SUMMER WITH THIS LOWFAT WINNER.

Ingredients

2 papayas, ripe
1 cup crushed pineapple
2 bananas, ripe

Directions

1. Blend all ingredients til smooth.
2. Chill in metal container until almost solid, about 3-4 hours.
3. Remove from freezer and blend.
4. Pour into individual serving dishes, cover, and chill for another 15-20 minutes.
5. Leave out for 5 minutes before serving.
6. Serves four.

Suggestion

This sorbet can also be made in an ice cream maker.

Pumpkin Pudding

A NUTRITIOUS VERSION OF AN ALL TIME FAVORITE TASTE.

Ingredients

4 cups Kabocha pumpkin(or Acorn squash), steamed and mashed (about 1 lg or 2 small pumpkins)
4 egg whites (or 2 eggs)
2 6oz pkgs vanilla soy malt
2 tsp cinnamon
1 tsp ginger
1/2 tsp nutmeg
1/2 cup almonds, slivered

Directions

1. Mix all ingredients, except almonds, until well-blended.
2. Toast almonds and fold into mixture.
3. Lightly oil a glass pie dish or 4 individual custard cups.
4. Pour in mixture and spread evenly.
5. Bake at 350 degrees F for 45 minutes or until set.
6. Serves four.

Suggestions

Serve topped with Tofu Vanilla Sauce (p. 133).
Use sweet potatoes or yams instead of pumpkin. Add 1/2 cup orange juice.

Pumpkins are rich in beta carotene.

Quinoa Pudding

ENJOY YOUR DESSERT WITH THIS ANCIENT STAPLE GRAIN OF THE ANDEAN CIVILIZATIONS.

Ingredients

1 1/2 cups water
1/2 cup quinoa, washed well
2 cups rice milk, soy milk, or amazake rice drink
1/2 tsp cardomon, crushed
1/2 tsp vanilla
2 tbsp blackstrap molasses
2 tbsp kuzu
2 tbsp water
1/2 cup Brazil nuts, chopped

Directions

1. Bring water to a boil.
2. Add quinoa and reduce heat.
3. Simmer, covered, for 15 minutes or until water is absorbed.
4. Add rice milk, cardomom, vanilla, and blackstrap molasses.
5. Simmer for another 5 minutes to allow flavors to blend.
6. Dissolve kuzu in water.
7. Add to mixture and cook, stirring frequently, for about 2-3 minutes or until thickened.
8. Pour into individual serving dishes and sprinkle with Brazil nuts.
9. Chill and serve.
10. Serves four.

Blackstrap molasses is an excellent source of iron and calcium.

Figgy Pudding

IN MEMORY OF CHRISTMAS PAST.

Ingredients

2 6 oz pkg vanilla soy malt
3-4 tbsp maple syrup (optional)
2 tbsp agar agar flakes
1 lb soft tofu
1 tsp cinnamon
4-6 Calimyrna figs, dried and snipped (or other figs of your choice)
1/3 cup chopped nuts
Nutmeg

Directions

1. Mix soy malt and agar agar flakes.
2. Heat over low flame till thickened.
3. Blend tofu and maple syrup.
4. Mix in soy malt mixture and cinnamon.
5. Fold in figs and nuts.
6. Pour into individual serving dishes and sprinkle with nutmeg.
7. Chill and serve.
8. Serves four.

Suggestions

For a sweeter pudding, add blackstrap molasses to taste.

Dried figs are a source of calcium.

Tropical Rice Pudding

A FRESH, LIGHT TASTE FROM THE ISLANDS.

Ingredients

1 1/2 cups brown rice, well-cooked
2 cups rice or soy milk
1 ripe banana, chopped or mashed
1/2 cup pineapple juice concentrate
1/2 cup pineapple chunks

Directions

1. In nonstick pan or double boiler, simmer first four ingredients for 30-45 minutes, or until pudding thickens.
2. Fold in pineapple chunks, chill, and serve.
3. Serves four.

Apricot Couscous Pie

HAVE YOUR PIE AND STAY HEALTHY TOO!

Ingredients

1 1/2 cups whole wheat couscous
2 cups soy milk
1/4 cup maple syrup
1/2 cup almonds (or other nuts) coarsely ground
1 1/2 cups apricot nectar
3 tbsp kuzu
10-15 apricots (or 10-15 dried, soaked overnight), chopped
1/4 tsp nutmeg
2-3 tbsp maple syrup (optional)

Directions

1. Bring couscous, soy milk, and maple syrup to a boil.
2. Lower flame and cook, covered, for 3-5 minutes. Remove from stove and let stand for 10 minutes until all liquid is absorbed.
3. Fluff with a fork and mix in nuts.
4. Dissolve kuzu in apricot nectar.
5. Bring nectar, apricots, and maple syrup to a boil.
6. Lower flame and cook for 2-3 minutes until thickened.
7. Stir constantly to avoid lumping.
8. In glass dish, pat down couscous mixture.
9. Top with apricot sauce.
10. Chill and serve.
11. Serves six.

Fresh Strawberry Delight

A QUICK, SIMPLE WAY TO ENJOY THE BERRIES OF THE SEASON.

Ingredients

1 lb fresh strawberries
1 cup nonfat plain yogurt
1 tsp vanilla
2-3 tbsp maple syrup

Directions

1. Wash strawberries and remove stems.
2. Place in individual serving dishes.
3. Mix yogurt, vanilla, and maple syrup till smooth.
4. Spoon over strawberries and serve.

Suggestions

If strawberries are extra large, keep stems on and use yogurt sauce as a dip.

Carob Cream Pie

THIS IS A RATHER RICH DESSERT TO BE SERVED ON SPECIAL OCCASIONS.

Ingredients

1 lb tofu, drained
1/3 cup maple syrup
1 tbsp canola oil
2 tsp vanilla
1/4 cup carob powder
1 prepared pie crust, whole wheat or graham cracker
1 banana, sliced

Directions

1. Slice tofu and press between layers of paper towel to remove excess water.
2. Blend tofu, maple syrup, oil, vanilla, and carob powder til smooth.
3. Pour into pie crust and decorate with banana slices.
4. Chill and serve.

Carob supplies the body with calcium.

Munchies

THE BEST BETWEEN MEAL SNACK IS FRESH, ORGANIC FRUIT. I ALSO KEEP THE FOLLOWING ON HAND TO APPEASE THE "MUNCHIE" CRAVINGS.

Dried figs, unsulphured

Dried apricots, unsulphured

Almonds

Raisins

Pumpkin seeds, unsalted

Sunflower seeds, unsalted

Popcorn (airpop and season with tamari and/or brewer's yeast) Spray with a small amount of olive oil.

A Final Note

As each person's constitution is different, individual needs will vary. I hope this book has given you some ideas so that you can refine your diet to meet your specific nutritional requirements.

In addition to a healthy diet, good digestion is a necessity for optimum health. Even the highest quality nutrients will do you no good if they are not absorbed and assimilated. Food allergies and sensitivities could also be a problem you may not be aware of. Over time, these allergies may result in disease. A nutritionally oriented physician or health practitioner can assist you with these issues and provide guidance in supplementing your diet based on your individual needs.

For good health and vibrant energy, regular progressive exercise is a necessity rather than a luxury. Weight-bearing, stretching, and walking, (or other cardiovascular exercise), will help keep bones strong and muscles toned.

Peace of mind is also a key factor in maintaining optimum health. Find whatever method of relaxation and stress release works for you and do it regularly.

Remember that learning to properly care for your body's needs is a gradual process. Be patient and persistent. Sooner or later you will begin to see results.

The human body is an amazing mechanism. Provide it with proper nutrition, regular exercise, and peace of mind, and it will respond magnificently.

Tips

- For reduced fat, sauté with 1/3 cup vegetable broth. Add water or additional broth as needed.
- For added iron, use a cast iron skillet.
- For reduced gas, soak beans overnight. Drain. Boil for 10 minutes. Drain again. Cook with a piece of kombu seaweed.
- For added calcium, soak washed egg shells in apple cider vinegar for up to six weeks (the longer the better). Remove egg shells and use vinegars in salads and as a condiment (Weed 192).
- For a fluffier basmati rice with separated grains, use 1 1/2 cups water to every 1 cup rice. Wrap lid with a towel to prevent steam from escaping.
- For a more nutritional dough, use organic whole grain flour, or a combination of flours, and make your own dough using the dough setting on your bread machine (if you happen to have one). You can also make the dough by hand if you are feeling ambitious.
- For a heart-healthy spread, add a sprig of fresh rosemary to a cup of extra virgin olive oil. Pour into a shallow container and refrigerate until solidified. Spread on bread and toast instead of margarine or butter.

Glossary

Aduki (Adzuki or Azuki) bean: A small red bean popular in Japan.

Agar Agar: A gelatinous substance from a sea vegetable.

Amazake: A nutritious drink made from sweet rice.

Arame: A sea vegetable that looks like tangled black strings. It is rather mild tasting in addition to being rich in calcium and iron.

Basmati rice: An aromatic rice from India, now also grown in the United States. Basmati rice is used in Ayurvedic nutritional healing.

Bok Choy: An oriental leafy green vegetable with thick, white stems.

Bragg liquid aminos: A sauce derived from soy beans that is naturally salty, yet contains far less sodium than table salt. Bragg also contains beneficial amino acids.

Burdock: A dark brown, long root that is very strengthening to the body.

Also called "gobo".

Fava bean: A broad bean that looks similar to a lima bean. Although fresh beans are seasonally available, dried beans can normally be found in natural food stores and Middle Eastern markets.

Feta: A white Greek cheese made from goat or ewe milk. Rinse before using to reduce salt.

Hijiki: A brown seaweed with a mild, nutty flavor. It looks like tangled black strings. It is high in calcium and other minerals.

Jasmine Rice: An aromatic rice popular in Thai cooking. Good for rice balls and sushi as it becomes moist and sticky when cooked.

Kashi: A brand name for a cereal made from seven whole grains.

Kelp: A generic name used for a variety of brown seaweeds. Kelp is rich in iodine, calcium, and other minerals. Kelp can be used as a condiment in place of salt, or taken in tablet form.

Kombu: A dark green sea vegetable that grows in deep waters. When cooked with beans, it aids in their digestion. Kombu also helps remove heavy metals from the body.

Kuzu (Kudzu): A white starch derived from a root by the same name. Rich in minerals, especially iron, it is used for thickening sauces and puddings.

Lavosh (Lahvosh or Thin Thin Bread): A wheat flat bread from the Middle East. Now available in natural food stores in addition to Middle Eastern markets.

Meatless sausage is made primarily from okara and spices, and it is cholesterol free. Morningstar Farms Links are a delicious choice, available in the freezer section of your local supermarket. Other varieties can be purchased at natural food stores.

Mirin: A cooking wine made from sweet rice. Used in Japanese cooking.

Miso paste is made from fermented soy beans and is the base of miso soup, a mainstay in Japan. Miso paste comes in dark and light varieties, with mild to strong flavors. Although salty, it has much less sodium than table salt. Highly nutritious, miso contains live enzymes that aid digestion. Miso should never be boiled.

Nutritional yeast, available in natural food stores, is a superior source of B-complex vitamins. It is also rich in organic iron and other minerals.

Rice Milk: A milk-like beverage made from brown rice.

Rice Vinegar: A vinegar derived from rice. Used in Oriental cooking.

Saffron: A fragrant yellow spice available in some supermarkets and Indian food stores. Saffron is cooling, tonifying, and aids digestion.

Seitan is a textured meat substitute made from wheat gluten boiled in a broth with tamari and kombu. It is a rich source of protein, yet low in fat.

Sesame Tahini is a nut butter made from sesame seeds. It can be found in supermarkets and natural food stores. Tahini is a rich source of calcium.

Shiitake Mushrooms: A mushroom known since ancient times for its numerous healing properties. Usually available dried, although fresh mushrooms can also be found in some parts of the country.

Soba: A Japanese noodle made from wheat and buckwheat flour.

Soy Milk: A milk-like beverage derived from soy.

Tamari is a wheat-free soy sauce readily available in most supermarkets.

Tempeh is made from fermented soybeans and is used as a source of protein.

Tofu: A curd made from soy beans. Takes on the flavor of whatever it is cooked with. Frozen and thawed, it has a "meaty" texture.

Tumeric is a yellow, aromatic root that lends color to soups and stews.

Tumeric aids in the digestion of protein. Purchase fresh when available.

Umeboshi: Small, red, pickled plums used in Japanese cooking. Umeboshi help stimulate digestion and keep the blood alkaline.

Vegetable Broth: A tasty broth made from vegetable bouillon and hot water. Vegetable bouillon is available in cube or bulk form at most natural food stores.

BIBLIOGRAPHY

Airola, Paavo. *Every Woman's Book*. Phoenix: Health Plus, 1979

Airola, Paavo. *How to Get Well*. Sherwood: Health Plus, 1974

Appleton, Nancy. *Healthy Bones*. Garden City Park: Avery Publishing Group, 1991

Balch, James F. et. al. *Prescription for Nutritional Healing*. Garden City Park: Avery Publishing Group, 1991

Boston Women's Health Book Collective, The. *The New Our Bodies, Ourselves*. New York: Touchstone, 1992

Carper, Jean. *Food - Your Miracle Medicine*. New York: Harper Perennial, 1993

Colgan, Michael. *Your Personal Vitamin Profile*. New York: Quill, 1982

Gardner, Joy. *The New Healing Yourself*. Freedom. The Crossing Press, 1989

Gittleman, Ann Louise. *Super Nutrition for Menopause*. New York: Pocket Books, 1993

Gittleman, Ann Louise. *Super Nutrition for Women*. New York: Bantam Books, 1991

Gladstar, Rosemary. *Herbal Healing for Women*. New York: Simon & Schuster, 1993

Grieve, M. *A Modern Herbal. Vol. I & II.* New York: Dover Publications, 1971

Haas, Elson. *Staying Healthy with the Seasons.* Berkely: Celestial Arts, 1981

Hausman, Patricia. *The Right Dose: How to Take Vitamins & Minerals Safely.* New York: Ballantine Books, 1987

Kushi, Michio. *The Quick and Natural Macrobiotic Cookbook.* Chicago: Contemporary Books, 1989

Lark, Susan M. *The Menopause Self Help Book.* Berkely: Celestial Arts, 1990

Morningstar, Amadea. *The Ayurvedic Cookbook.* Santa Fe: Lotus Press, 1990

Rose, Jeanne. *Jeanne Rose's Herbal Guide to Food.* Berkely: North Atlantic Books, 1979

Santillo, Humbart. *Natural Healing with Herbs.* Prescott: Hohm Press, 1989

Shook, Edward E. *Elementary Treatise in Herbology.* Banning: Enos Publishing Company, 1993

Somer, Elizabeth. *Nutrition for Women.* New York: Henry Holt and Company, 1993

Tierra, Michael. *Planetary Herbology.* Santa Fe: Lotus Press, 1988

Tierra, Michael. *The Way of Herbs.* New York: Pocket Books, 1980

Ulene, Art. *Nutrition Facts Desk Reference.* Garden City Park: Avery Publishing Group, 1995

Weed, Susan S. *Menopausal Years: The Wise Woman Way.* Woodstock: Ash Tree Publishing, 1992

Williams, Jude C. *Jude's Herbal Home Remedies.* St. Paul: Llewellyn Publications, 1994

Wright, Jonathan V. *Dr. Wright's Guide to Healing Nutrition.* New Canaan: Keats Publishing, 1984